The Practice of Natural Childbirth

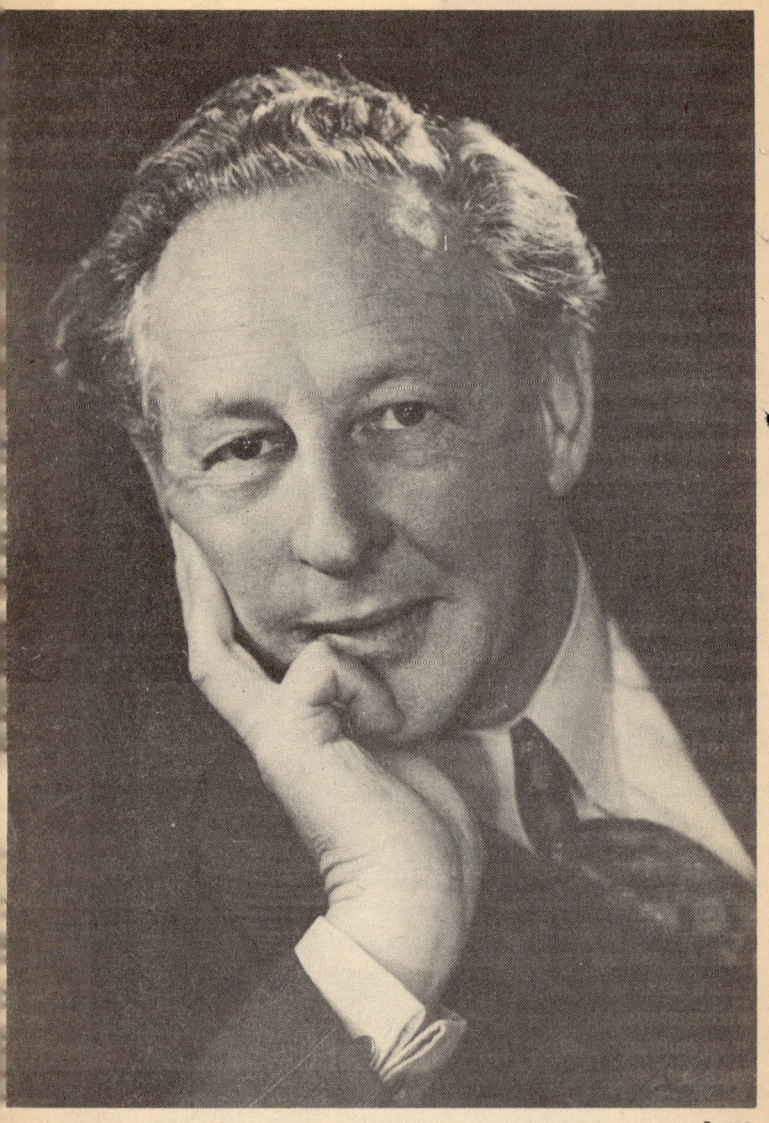

Grantly Dick-Read, M.D.

Prager

The Practice of
NATURAL CHILDBIRTH

Grantly Dick-Read, M.D.

Revised and Edited by
Helen Wessel and Harlan F. Ellis, M.D.

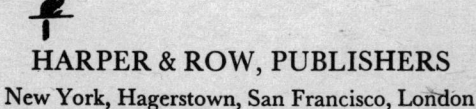

HARPER & ROW, PUBLISHERS
New York, Hagerstown, San Francisco, London

This book is one of three sections of *Childbirth Without Fear: The Original Approach to Natural Childbirth,* New Fourth Edition, also published by Harper & Row, Publishers.

Copyright 1944, 1953 by Grantly Dick-Read. Renewed 1972 by Jessica Dick-Read Bennett. Copyright © 1959, 1972 by Jessica Dick-Read. All rights reserved. Printed in the United States of America. No part of this book may be used or reproduced in any manner without written permission except in the case of brief quotations embodied in critical articles and reviews. For information address Harper & Row, Publishers, Inc., 10 East 53d Street, New York, N.Y. 10022. Published simultaneously in Canada by Fitzhenry & Whiteside Limited, Toronto.

First BARNES & NOBLE BOOKS edition published 1976

ISBN: 0-06-465049-9

77 78 79 80 5 4 3

Contents

Foreword xiii

1. **Prenatal Health** 1
   Diet
   Clothing
   Personal Hygiene

2. **Education** 6
   Fertilization
   Development of the Human Baby
   The Uterus During Pregnancy
   The Muscle Layers of the Uterus
   Fear-Tension-Pain
   Hospital Tour

3. **Breathing** 16
   Full Deep Breathing
   "Work" Breathing
   "Sleep" Breathing
   Breath-holding
   Rapid Breathing

4. **Relaxation** 22
   Preparation for Relaxation
   Recognizing Tension
   Practicing Relaxation
   Breathing
   Positions for Relaxation
   Residual Tension

5. **Physical Fitness** 38
   Posture
   Exercises
   Pelvic Rock
   Squatting, with variations

CONTENTS

Firming the Breasts
Labor Position
Firming Pelvic Floor Muscles

6. Labor (First-Stage Labor) 50
   Onset of Labor
   Early First-Stage Labor
   Late First-Stage Labor
   Position
   Breathing
   Relaxation
   Discomfort
   Transition
   Summary of First-Stage Labor

7. Birth (Second-Stage Labor) 65
   Early Second-Stage Labor
   The Husband
   Position
   Well-Established Second-Stage Labor
   Breathing
   Relaxation
   Anesthesia
   Birth
   Summary of Second-Stage Labor

8. Immediate Newborn Period (Third-Stage Labor) 79
   Addendum: Instructions on the Immediate Routine
             Care of the Newborn

9. Natural Childbirth in Emergency 88

10. Care of the Newborn 94
    Body Contact
    Colostrum
    Feeding on Demand
    Baby's Perfect Food
    Rooming-In
    Addendum: Infant Care in the Nursery
              Suggested Rooming In Procedures

11. **The New Mother** 105
    Afterpains
    Lochia
    Care of the Nipples
    Breastfeeding
    Rooming-In
    Diet
    Postnatal Exercises
       Breathing
       Firming Pelvic Floor
       Firming Abdominal Muscles
       Firming the Breasts
       Pelvic Rock
       Conclusion

Illustrations

        GRANTLY DICK-READ FRONTISPIECE
16. Full-term infant in uterus   10
17–19. Muscle layers of the uterus   13
20–21. Quiet diaphragmatic breathing   19
22–23. Learning relaxation   28
24–25. Husband checking relaxation   29
26. Reclining chair position   34
27–28. Relaxing in left lateral position   34, 35
29. Husband checking relaxation   35
30–31. Relaxation in pregnancy and labor   36
32–33. Pelvic rocking   42
34. Squatting   43
35–36. Squatting, variation a   43
37–38. Squatting, variations b, c   44
39. Sitting Indian style   45
40. Firming the breasts   45
41–42. Second-stage pushing, practice and real   46
43–44. Second-stage resting, practice and real   47
45–46. Arrival at hospital in labor   52
47–49. First-stage labor   55
50–53. In labor with twins   57
54–56. Early second-stage in labor room   67
57. Husband scrubbing before accompanying wife to birth room   69
58. Accompanying wife to birth room   69
59. Resting against backrest in birth room (in labor with twins)   69
60. Bearing down in second-stage labor   71
61. Resting between contractions   71
62. Baby's head born   77
63. Baby's body emerges   77
64. Physician showing baby to mother   81
65. Proud parents admiring newborn   81

ILLUSTRATIONS

66. Physician showing placenta   83
67. Physician showing membranes   83
68. Twins!   85
69. Walking to room after giving birth to twins   85
70–72. Skin-to-skin contact   96, 97

Gary Davis of Fireside Photos was the photographer for the photos contained herein.

The Practice of Natural Childbirth

Foreword

It has been over fifty years since Grantly Dick-Read (1890–1959) first prepared a monograph on his carefully developed philosophy of childbirth. At that time, the concept of childbirth as a positive experience, free from suffering, was a shocking and revolutionary idea, unacceptable to many, for almost all women in labor were delivered under deep anesthesia.

At the height of his successful obstetric practice, at forty years of age, he wrote a book that was to change the course of obstetric history. He had proven from his own experiences as a physician his belief that childbirth is a natural physiological process not meant to be painful, and because he had built his teaching around a study of the "laws of nature," he chose for his book the title *Natural Childbirth*. He had not the faintest notion that this book title would be taken as a "name" for this kind of childbirth experience! Indeed, though often misunderstood, the term became a household word everywhere, for when the book was published in 1933, Grantly Dick-Read rose from the relative obscurity of a local medical practice into a target for the ire or praise of people all over the world.

Later his teachings were incorporated in a larger book called *Childbirth Without Fear,* first published in the United States in 1944 by Harper and Row, currently in its fourth edition.

The following chapters on The Practice of Natural Childbirth are taken from this fourth edition. They contain specific instructions for the successful application of Grantly Dick-Read's natural childbirth principles.

The emphasis throughout his teaching is always upon naturalness, upon that which is most easily learned, practiced, and applied. The reader will discover that all the techniques he advocates one practice during pregnancy for comfortable childbearing are simple, everyday rules of good health. *Disciplined practice of these few basic techniques is essential for a happy outcome at birth.*

Grantly Dick-Read did not envision his teaching on childbirth as an "end" to discovery, but as a true foundation from which many further discoveries could be made, although to date there has been nothing added in the way of "new techniques" for comfortable childbirth that substantially improves upon his method, or that invalidates his teaching when correctly applied.

If he were with us today he would encourage us to keep on asking questions, to keep on challenging tradition, to keep on testing current medical practices and theories, including his own, for validity. All those who share his faith in the consistency and orderliness of natural law, which we disregard at our own peril, will continue in the search for truth.

HELEN WESSEL
HARLAN ELLIS, M.D.

1975

1

Prenatal Health

The general hygiene of pregnancy often brings to light much that surprises. Too many women of all income classes are ignorant of habits and customs they should have learned and practiced from early childhood. Women must associate the necessity for care of their own health with the health of their unborn babies.

DIET

There is little reason why a woman should alter the normal diet with which she has maintained good health. Her body is accustomed to it, and any sudden change may do more harm than good. It is well that she eat slightly less than usual, but skipping meals or going on crash diets to avoid weight gain is foolish, and detrimental to her basic health and vitality.

The Victorian idea that a pregnant woman eats for two people must also be dispelled. Excessive eating during pregnancy is even more harmful than at other times. If a woman is excessively fat, she should follow a carefully balanced diet prepared for her by her own physician, and under his constant supervision.

Vegetarians need not add to or change their food. They generally have less trouble with pregnancy and labor than those who are heavy meat-eaters, because the latter tend to skimp on fresh vegetables and fruits. If a woman is accustomed to eating meat, she would do well to choose liver, fish, and poultry more often than beef, pork, or lamb, and to balance it with salads rather than potatoes and gravy.

Fluids assist in the metabolism of other foods. An adequate amount of *protein* is essential, and is found in lean meat, eggs, milk, peas, beans, and nuts. Wheat germ is an excellent source of added protein and B vitamins. *Fats* are necessary as fuel for heat and energy in the body, and are obtained in cream, butter, cheese, and some of the fat meats. *Carbohydrates* are also energy making, and are supplied in sweets, flour, sugar, potatoes, milk, and rice. Unrefined natural sugars are probably the best source of carbohydrates.

Iron, calcium, phosphorus, iodine, and other *minerals* and *vitamins* are all necessary, and are supplied in a well-balanced diet containing fish and liver, milk, grains (100 percent whole wheat, barley, oats, etc.), vegetables, and fresh citrus fruits. Vitamin and mineral tablets as diet supplements are not necessary, unless the physician diagnoses some particular deficiency. Alcohol is best kept to a minimum, and smoking is not advisable.

CLOTHING

Psychologically, clothing has a much greater influence than is generally recognized. An expectant mother should look attractive, wearing suitable clothes, without trying to hide her shape or feel embarrassed by it. For her own composure she should realize that sensible people envy and admire a young pregnant woman.

After the first two or three months of pregnancy the center of gravity alters, so that it is safer to wear low heels. Many pregnant women fall downstairs or trip easily for no apparent reason, and although the majority of these accidents do no harm to either mother or baby, they are disconcerting and cause unnecessary anxiety.

After the fourth month there must be no undue pressure on the abdomen. Dresses and smocks should hang from the shoulders, and skirts and slacks should be adjustable to the changing shape of the body.

The breasts should be supported within well-fitting, rounded cups, with straps that lift them to the correct height upon the chest, but without any pressure whatever across the breasts or nipples.

Abdominal supporting belts are rarely required by a woman having her first baby, and those who have carried out their prenatal and postnatal exercises in order to maintain the tone of abdominal muscles do not require them for subsequent babies. But when a support is necessary, the general principle is that the uterus should be supported from below in a cup-shaped garment, with no pressure whatever on it above the level of the navel. Such a support helps keep the uterus from falling forward, and relieves backache by taking the weight of the developing uterus from the muscles in the small of the back.

PERSONAL HYGIENE

The Skin

It is not unusual, particularly for brunettes, to develop large areas of brown pigment on the forehead or cheekbones, or on other parts of the body. There is no way of preventing or curing this, but it does tend to disappear after pregnancy.

Sometimes itching is troublesome, probably due to stretching of the tissues. This can be relieved by keeping the skin clean and soft with a good alkaline soap or one of the many creams available for this purpose. Itching of the genitals arises from different causes, and should be reported to the doctor for his advice on treatment.

The Hair

During pregnancy there is sometimes a tendency for the hair to become rather lifeless, and to fall out. The hair should be given a good brushing, and a few drops of thin hair oil or lotion should be rubbed into the scalp. The chances are, if nutrition is adequate and the hair washed as often as is necessary, this bit of extra attention will help it keep its vitality and look better after pregnancy than before.

Fingernails

Fingernails can be kept from cracking by rubbing a little vaseline on and around them at night. To keep from harming the baby after its arrival, the nails should be kept short and clean.

The Teeth

As soon as a woman knows she is pregnant, she should have a thorough examination made of her mouth by a dentist, to see that no decay or sepsis is present. The teeth do tend to decay more while a baby is coming, due to the changes in a woman's own system, and not because of the baby's need for calcium. During pregnancy many women also tend to get red and puffy gums, which may bleed easily. A very soft tooth brush should be used and the gums massaged. This problem will disappear shortly after the baby is born.

The Breasts and Nipples

The nipples should be kept clean with warm water during the daily bath or shower, but no soap or other product whatever should be used on them. The softer and more elastic the nipples can be kept, the better for the woman who wishes to breastfeed her baby.

During the last ten or twelve weeks of pregnancy the breasts may exude a few drops of a very thick, yellow secretion called *colostrum*. If it cakes on the breasts, warm water will soften it, and, if it gets too thick, very gentle pressure at the base of the nipple with the thumb and forefinger will clear the little openings into the breast. This should be done extremely gently and without any force at all. Great care should be taken that the breasts are never handled roughly, or violently rubbed or massaged, as some erroneously advise.

If the nipple is slightly retracted and doesn't stand out as it should after warm bathing, this should be called to the attention of the doctor. He may advise wearing a breast shield during pregnancy to help the nipple come forward, so the baby will be able to nurse more easily later.

The Bowels

A glass of hot water, with or without a teaspoonful of honey stirred into it, helps maintain a daily bowel action when taken first thing in the morning. If constipation is a problem, stewed prunes, raw apples, figs, or raisins eaten with breakfast are helpful. No other tablets or preparations should be taken unless a doctor so advises.

2

Education

The human body is not a series of individual organs carrying out their allotted tasks unaffected by their neighbors. Our bodies are unified structures whose components exhibit the most perfect harmony that science has the privilege of investigating. Our organs and purposes are interdependent. No physical strain beyond our ability can be sustained without circulatory or skeletal injury, and no chronic fear or anxiety can be maintained in the human mind without the disruption of the normal physiological balance. The manifestations of such fear or anxiety may be either psychological or physical, for nature rebels against intruders upon its ordered processes.

It is important for women to understand the development of a baby within the uterus, for ignorance of these elementary facts may cause anxieties and doubts that are difficult to overcome, affecting her health adversely. Such complaints of pregnancy as persistent nausea, sickness, constipation, desire for unusual foods, excessive salivation, headaches, backaches, and a general feeling of weariness, may often be the physical manifestations of anxiety, which knowledge can help dispel.

FERTILIZATION

Nearly all animals, including human beings, have much the same principles of breeding. The female makes eggs and the male produces sperm. Eggs have to be fertilized by the sperm before they can grow into babies. Nature makes the process of fertilization pleasant to experience, because each race must go on reproducing itself or it will die out.

The female reproductive organs are located in the lower abdomen, below the level of the hip bones. In the center of these is the *uterus,* or womb, which in its nonpregnant state is about two and one-half inches by one and one-half inches by one-half inch. A small, muscular organ that weighs about one and one-half ounces, the uterus is shaped rather like a pear with the narrow end pointing downward, where it is attached to the upper end of the vagina. The lower, narrow end of the uterus is closed by circular muscular tissue called the *cervix,* through which a narrow passage opens into the uterus.

At the upper end of the uterus are two narrow tubes that extend out from each side, rather like arms extending out from the shoulders. Each tube is three or four inches long, and opens at the end furthest from the uterus into a shallow bell shape. Underneath each of these two bell-shaped structures is a small, oval organ called an *ovary.* Each of the two ovaries contain *ova,* or egg-forming tissue.

An egg (*ovum*) is developed and sent on its way by one of the ovaries each month, about ten days after menstruation. The ovum travels down the narrow tube from the ovary to the uterus, while the uterus prepares a lining of tissue to make a good "nest" to receive it. If the egg is not fertilized by a male sperm, it passes on through the uterus and is cast off. About two weeks later the lining of the uterus is also thrown off, and a new lining prepared for the next egg. The flow of cast-off, unused material is called *menstruation.*

A male child is born with testicles which, shortly before birth, have moved down from the abdomen into the scrotum, outside the body. In these organs *spermatozoa* are produced. It is estimated that each testicle contains over one mile of sperm-producing tubules, from the walls of which a healthy man may produce at each ejaculation over two hundred million spermatozoa.

The male sperm is ejaculated from the penis into the vagina of the female at the culmination of mating, or *coitus.* The mature sperm cell has a long, thin tail, which enables it to move toward the opening in the cervix of the uterus. It travels at the rate of about one inch in ten minutes. Considerable numbers find their way into the uterus and engage in what might be described as a race for the ovum. As soon as a sperm penetrates an ovum, making it fertile, the ovum undergoes an immediate change, which prevents any further penetration by another sperm.

The fertile egg moves on through the tube, becomes embedded in the wall of the uterus, and starts to grow. The lining of the uterus alters its character, developing the *placenta,* through which the mother nourishes her child. The placental site rapidly expands, its blood vessels and nerve fibrils bring vitality to the egg, and the growth of the *fetus,* the developing baby, begins.

DEVELOPMENT OF THE HUMAN BABY

Very shortly after the ovum is fertilized it starts to develop cells that are differentiated to form the various organs and structures of the body. Some of these become the mother cells of spermatozoa and ova, so that quite early in fetal life the sex of the child is determined.

During its growing life, the baby is protected by a "bag of waters," in which it lives. This protects the baby from injury if the mother is bumped or falls, keeps him or her at a constant temperature, and provides space for the baby to move about freely until the later months of growth.

The fetus grows very fast. At four weeks it is one sixth of an inch long, lying in a fluidlike sack about the size of a pigeon's egg. At the end of the second month it is about one and one-sixth inches long, and the arms, legs, and head are clearly distinguishable. By this time it has its own circulation of blood and its own nervous system.

It is now fed through its navel by a tube called the *umbilical cord,* which is attached to the placenta. This wonderful organ, the placenta, is attached to the inside wall of the uterus and filters from the mother's blood the substances necessary for the development of the child. Not only does it have the power of passing on to the child what it requires, but it also has the power of refusing to take from the mother's blood some of the substances that may not be advantageous to the child. By the time the baby is due to be born, the umbilical cord between the placenta and baby may be from one to three feet in length.

At the end of the third month the fetus is about three and one-half inches long, weighs approximately an ounce, and at the end of the fourth month it has grown rapidly to about seven inches and weighs about four ounces. Its heart can now be heard beating strongly, and it is possible to tell the sex of the child if it should be born at this stage. By this time the mother will have become conscious of the baby's movements. This is known as *quickening,* and it occurs at about eighteen or nineteen weeks after conception.

Out of all proportion to the skeletal growth of the baby is the development of its brain. From the earliest weeks, brain substance is present in the fetus. At three and a half weeks the brain can be differentiated into its three main divisions, and between three and five months it develops integrative cerebral function. One month before the baby is born its brain is perfected.

It is within the brain itself that the heritage of parental influence is most readily discovered. The baby's mental development is influenced, not only by heredity, but also by the nature of the mother's influence during pregnancy. The calmness or anxiety that affects her own nervous system may have an effect on the baby also.

At the fifth month of pregnancy the baby is almost ten inches long and weighs about one and one-half pounds. Occasionally one reads in medical literature of babies born at this age who survive. By the end of the seventh month, twenty-eight weeks old, the child is perfected. Although not fully grown or fully nourished, some twenty-eight-week-old children have survived well after birth.

At the eighth month the child is almost seventeen inches

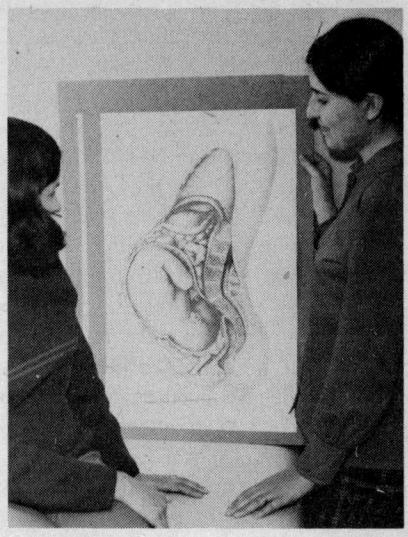

Fig. 16. Instructor showing patient diagram of baby at full term.

long, and has a very good chance of healthy survival. At the ninth month, or thirty-six weeks, the average weight is five to five and one-half pounds. The organs and functions are all well developed, and although children born now require more care than full-term children, they should survive perfectly well if born at this age.

At the tenth month, forty weeks—which is about the average time a child takes to develop—it should weigh about seven to seven and one-half pounds and be about nineteen inches in length (fig. 16), and it is in this condition that natural birth takes place.

THE UTERUS DURING PREGNANCY

The duration of pregnancy is counted from the first day of the last menstrual period. Most women suspect that they are pregnant when the expected period does not arrive. They feel perfectly well, unless for any reason they are anxious about pregnancy. When about six or seven weeks pregnant, many women will be conscious of sensitiveness and slight enlargement of the breasts. By this time the pregnant woman should see a doctor, and keep in constant touch with him or a clinic throughout the whole of pregnancy, and until at least six weeks after the birth of the baby. These chapters are not intended to instruct mothers in matters that are the special province of medical advisers. There must be someone qualified to whom they can turn for advice upon any subject that creates the slightest doubt in their minds.

With the growth of the fetus the uterus develops in size. The muscle fibers become longer and more numerous. Fluid is secreted into the cavity of the organ, which fills and expands. After two months the pregnant uterus is about the size of a large hen's egg. At the third month it can just be felt, in a thin woman, above the pubic bone. At the fourth month it is halfway between the pubic bone and the navel. At five and a half months it is up to the navel. At eight months it is about halfway between the navel and the lower end of the breastbone.

Between the seventh and eighth month the baby's heart beats loudly enough for the mother to hear it through the doctor's stethoscope, although the doctor, with his practiced ear, will have been able to detect it long before this time.

By thirty-five weeks the baby should have taken up its correct position for birth, with its head downward and its back slightly to the right or the left of center. At nine and a half months, or thirty-eight weeks, the uterus reaches its highest point in the abdomen.

At about the thirty-eighth week women who are having their first baby will experience what is known as *lightening*. This is the slipping down of the baby's head into the brim of the pelvis. The baby's chin becomes flexed upon his breastbone, and the back of his head (called the *occiput*) slides downward into the upper portion of the birth canal. The change is often felt in the abdomen. The uterus appears to have lowered, and this often gives the mother added freedom of movement and breathing. Thus at full term, or forty weeks, the uterus has dropped back one to two inches. The actual size of the uterus varies according to the amount of water in it and the size of the baby, but the levels in the abdomen at certain weeks of development do not vary much in different women.

The birth of the child may usually be expected within ten days or two weeks after this lightening occurs. With second and subsequent babies it may not occur, however. Not infrequently, in the easiest births of additional children, the head will remain quite high in the pelvis, or even above it, until well into the second stage of labor.

THE MUSCLE LAYERS OF THE UTERUS

When the baby is ready to be born, the uterus is a muscular bag about fourteen inches in length and not quite half an inch in thickness. It is well supplied with nerves that stimulate its muscles to contract, and it also has a plentiful supply of blood vessels, which are necessary to take fresh blood to the uterus and to carry away all the waste products of muscular activity. There are three muscle layers in the uterus (figs. 17–19):

1. The outer layer goes up the back, over the top, and down the front. These long muscle bands are found mainly in the middle and upper part of the uterus.

2. The middle muscle layer is a mass of interwoven muscles in which the big blood vessels lie.

3. The inner muscle layer goes around the uterus in a circular manner, and is found almost entirely in the area of the lower part of the uterus and cervix.

The outer muscles contract (shorten and tighten) to push the baby down, through, and ultimately out of the uterus. The middle muscles contract to squeeze the blood out of the walls of the uterus, and then relax to allow the blood vessels to fill up again with a fresh supply of blood.

But when the inner, circular muscles contract, they close the outlet, maintaining the uterus in its unemptied shape. Thus these inner, circular muscles *must be loose and relaxed* when

MUSCLES OF THE UTERUS

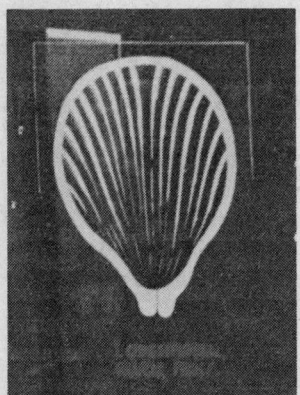

Fig. 17. Longitudinal muscle fibers.

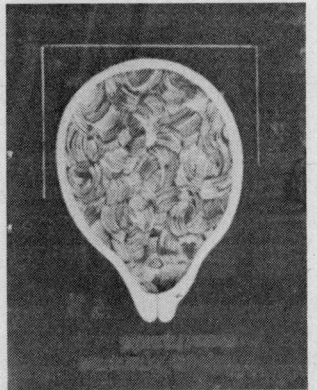

Fig. 18. Muscles interwoven with blood vessels.

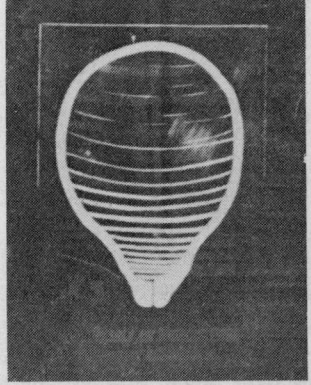

Fig. 19. Circular muscle fibers.

the long muscles contract to open the womb and push the baby out. If a woman is frightened during labor, this inner muscle layer contracts. Then the muscles that empty the uterus and the muscles that hold it closed are working against each other.

All through the body one finds examples of the harmony of muscles in polarity. For example, one's biceps relax when the triceps hold out the arm, but the triceps relax when the biceps pull the forearm up to the shoulder. If both sets of muscles are activated at the same time, pain soon results.

Whenever there are two big groups of muscles working against each other they soon begin to hurt, and in a short time the pain becomes very severe. We speak of this as the "fear-tension-pain syndrome" of childbirth, for a woman who is afraid is unconsciously resisting the birth of her baby by tightening the circular fibers, preventing the progress of the birth, and increasing the muscle tension within the walls of the uterus. This causes nearly all the pains and distresses in otherwise normal labor, which describes the labor of about ninety-five women out of a hundred.

FEAR-TENSION-PAIN

This fear-tension-pain series of events is experienced by everybody in circumstances very similar. The bowel is full, the desire to empty is acute, it pushes against our active restraint, but the time and place are not convenient. We are afraid to stop resisting even though it is uncomfortable and becoming painful, until there is the right opportunity to relax the outlet and let the contents be released. Again, we have a strong urge to urinate, but the right place is not available. We dare not relax the muscles that hold the bladder closed because of social and domestic repercussions, so we suffer increasing pain, sometimes agony, until the opportunity comes for the comfort of relaxing the outlet and emptying the distended, contracting organ.

This same principle is at work during the birth of a child. Fear of pain causes resistance to the working muscles of the uterus, increasing tension and causing pain. The muscles of the bowel and bladder are less powerful than those of the uterus, but even they become painful if their efforts to expel are resisted.

Fear is the natural protective emotion without which few of us would remain alive for many days. Its intensity varies from precaution and doubt to uncontrollable terror. Even mild anxiety can make a woman tense, thus causing the circular muscles to resist the expulsive muscles of the uterus. A tense woman has a tense outlet to the uterus, giving rise to the saying "Tense woman—tense cervix." A tense cervix means a long and painful labor in the majority of cases, for the mother is closing the door against the progress of her baby from the uterus.

By contrast, a relaxed woman allows the cervix, the "door" of the uterus, to open easily. If she understands what is taking place, is fully relaxed and confident, then the muscles that held the uterus closed during pregnancy will become loose and easily stretched open, when the long muscles begin their work of expelling the baby. The tension created by resistance to the birth will not be there to cause pain, and the baby will be born more easily and comfortably.

3

Breathing

The growth of the baby inside the uterus is maintained through the mother's blood. The wonderful organ known as the placenta, which develops along with the baby, is able to filter from the large blood vessels of the uterus the food required by the baby. This is passed to the baby through the umbilical cord to his navel. Through the cord the waste material of the baby is returned as well, to be disposed of by the mother. So it becomes clear that to have healthy babies it is necessary to eat and drink the right things.

One of the most important foods is oxygen. We cannot live without it, and whenever the supply of oxygen to the brain is insufficient for a short period of time, the brain becomes damaged to that degree. Adults breathe in oxygen through their lungs. The baby doesn't use its lungs for breathing, but takes its oxygen from the placenta straight into its bloodstream. Therefore, by breathing correctly, the mother can supply as much oxygen to her baby as it requires. During pregnancy it is of the utmost importance that as much fresh air as possible is taken into her lungs, and with the least effort.

Correct breathing is also essential during labor. The big muscles of the uterus are working to expel the baby, and when big muscles are used they require more fuel, just as a car uses more fuel to go faster or climb a hill. We don't feel our big muscles working if we are healthy, but we do breathe faster and deeper, and that is how they get extra fuel. During labor correct breathing is essential in supplying the necessary oxygen to the working muscles of the uterus. It also keeps the baby strong and in good condition while it is being born.

But in order for the breathing to help, the mother must also be *relaxed* enough during labor to allow the blood to circulate more freely through the middle layer of muscles in the uterus, thus replenishing its oxygen supply more quickly and plentifully.

No one can work to the best of her ability either physically or mentally if she does not breathe correctly; indeed, incorrect breathing is *the* bad habit that causes more illness than any other. It is surprising to learn that not one woman in fifty breathes properly.

The secret of correct breathing lies in the *control* of respiration—that is, control of breathing in and also of breathing out. Fresh air is taken into the lungs, which are like a very fine sponge made of minute air spaces and even smaller blood vessels. The walls are so thin that the oxygen from the air passes into the blood and the waste gas from the blood passes into the air spaces. By breathing we take in pure air and get rid of "waste" air.

Most people use less than four-fifths of their air space. To maintain a sufficient supply of oxygen, this means that they have to breathe five times for every four breaths taken by the person who breathes correctly. Breathing faster means more work for the muscles concerned with breathing, and more work for the heart to pump the blood around the body. In pregnancy this can become a strain and even a discomfort, the enlarging uterus causes discomfort to many women because they do not maintain good posture and breathe correctly. Therefore, during this time, when the oxygen intake is so dependent upon the correctness of breathing, these simple exercises should have priority over all other physical movements.

1. FULL DEEP BREATHING

Place your hands flat on your lower ribs, with your head up and shoulders back. Open your mouth and fill your chest slowly with air, filling in the upper part of the lungs as well as the lower, clear up under the collarbones. When you have breathed in as much air as possible, then let it out, slowly and completely. Lean slightly forward and force out the last possible breath. This will not cause any harm, so don't be afraid to take these slow, deep breaths.

Spend five or ten minutes each morning and evening breathing in and out, slowly and deeply, in this way. Many women are surprised at how much better they feel after only two weeks of practicing this simple breathing exercise each day. They quickly find themselves able to do more without becoming "out of breath." Rapid progress is made because there is usually so much room for improvement!

2. "WORK" BREATHING

When you have acquired the habit of freely breathing deeply, learn to breathe more quickly, but still keeping the breathing under control, while working around the house. Instead of seventeen or eighteen breaths a minute, gradually work up to *twenty-five or twenty-six times a minute,* but not faster. This "work" breathing supplies the extra oxygen needed for physical exertion, and is of great help in labor during the contractions near the end of the first stage. These in-and-out breaths, which are still to be taken deep into the diaphragm, should not be confused with shallow panting, which, since it tends to become too rapid, may lead to hyperventilation and may limit the oxygen supply to the uterus.

3. "SLEEP" BREATHING

Next, learn gentle diaphragmatic breathing, in a relaxed and comfortable position in a chair, or on the bed. This

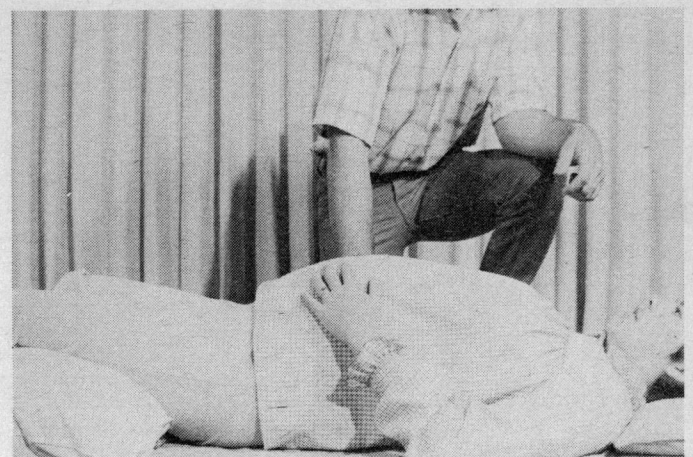

Fig. 20. Deep, quiet breathing—inhalation. Notice husband's watch is out of sight.

Fig. 21. Deep, quiet breathing—exhalation. Notice husband's watch.

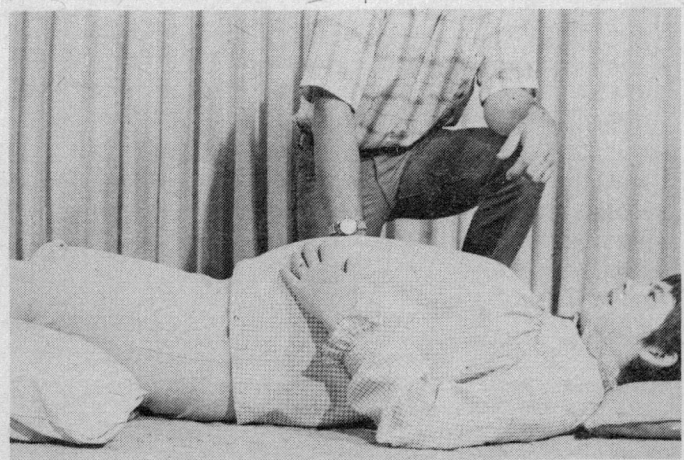

breathing is the normal breathing experienced in relaxed sleep, when an observer can see the lower diaphragm and the abdomen rising and falling gently.

Take a deep breath into the diaphragm, but not so deep that it also fills the upper chest. As the diaphragm gently expands, the abdomen can be seen rising (fig. 20). Slowly let the breath out again, letting the abdomen fall gently (fig. 21). After a few such slow, deep breaths, a person often yawns, showing that this breathing is a real aid to relaxation. As this quiet, slower breathing deep in the diaphragm is continued and the person becomes more relaxed, the breathing itself becomes automatic and no longer requires attention to continue.

This relaxed, natural "sleep" breathing is invaluable during pregnancy for falling asleep at night, and is most helpful in providing comfort during the first stage of labor by making relaxation more effective.

Some women push up the abdomen with its muscles while breathing in, but this is a mistake.* The abdominal muscles must stay completely slack, the abdominal wall rising and falling of its own accord as the air is taken deep into the diaphragm and released.

4. BREATH-HOLDING

Take one deep breath, let it all the way out; take another, let it all the way out. Then take a full breath and *hold it*. In your mind count up to ten, then let the air out through your mouth, not in a rush, but with control. After holding your breath, again take one or two deep in-and-out breaths to clear the lungs of stale air and replenish the oxygen supply. Practice

* Grantly Dick-Read's breathing technique is often confused with that of Helen Heardman, as outlined in her *Physiotherapy in Obstetrics-Gynecology* (Edinburgh: Livingstone, 1951). She taught a form of abdominal breathing in which the breath was held for long periods —one or two breaths a minute. This method is foreign to Dick-Read's approach! —Ed.

the breath-holding as the weeks go by until you experience no difficulty in holding a full breath for half a minute. (Remember, always take one or two deep in-and-out breaths both before and after holding the breath.)

Learning to hold the breath makes the work easier in the second stage of labor, when each contraction of the uterus needs you to hold your breath and push down to help the baby through the birth canal.

5. RAPID BREATHING

Learn to breathe short in-and-out breaths with the mouth open, but *not more than thirty-five to forty a minute*. This is necessary just as the baby is being born, since it keeps the mother from pushing down as the baby's head emerges slowly. It helps prevent any sudden and excessive pressure on the outlet, and thus helps avoid tearing its edges.

This more rapid breathing should be practiced just enough to learn how to do it. It is to be used in labor *only* to keep from bearing down, and under a doctor's continual supervision.

4

Relaxation

It is necessary for a woman carrying a baby to have a certain amount of rest, even if it is only for half an hour a day. Physical tiredness may become embarrassing in the later stages of pregnancy if the habit of rest is not acquired in the earlier months. Learning to relax properly makes this rest more effective.

Thus relaxation is of great benefit during pregnancy. Half an hour's relaxation is worth more than twice that time in sleep. It releases states of tension that a woman might unconsciously develop, and so helps avoid all manner of aches and pains. It introduces a calmness and helps establish confidence, which, in a state of tension, is practically impossible to do. Tension is caused by anxiety, and relaxation helps overcome anxiety by relieving tension of the mind as well as of the body.

Relaxation is also of the greatest possible assistance to a woman during labor. If she is able to become completely relaxed *during* the contractions of the first stage and *between* the contractions of the second stage, she will find that normal labor has no unbearable discomfort from beginning to end.

But relaxation is not only of value for pregnancy and labor. If it is continued, it lays a foundation for good health afterward also. We all live under considerable stress, and there is more emotional as well as physical weariness than is usually recognized. Such tension undermines both health and happiness in the rush of modern living. A woman who practices relaxation enhances her natural beauty, is more poised both with friends and with strangers, and is more at ease with her newborn and her husband.

The teaching of relaxation should be begun about the time that the mother is conscious of the quickening of her child. Most intelligent women can learn enough in the remaining months to enable them to get very good results in labor.

Muscular relaxation is a condition in which *the muscle tone throughout the body is reduced to a minimum*. When muscular tension is absent, emotional reactions and even thought patterns fade. Thus a completely slack body during labor eliminates any excess of muscle tone in the circular fibers of the lower uterine segment, the cervix, and the outlet of the birth canal. And this is not all. In a state of complete relaxation and mental calm, the sensations of uterine muscle activity during labor are interpreted in their true sense, just as the contraction of the biceps in the arm might be interpreted.

PREPARATION FOR RELAXATION

Draw the curtains and darken the room slightly—bright sunshine makes relaxation more difficult than shade or soft light. Before starting to relax, eyeglasses and dentures, if any, should be removed. The bladder must be completely empty so that the pelvic muscles can safely be relaxed.

It is important that the person relaxing be in such a comfortable position that she feels no need of support to remain in that position without moving. She should be on a very firm bed or couch or on the floor, with a folded blanket under her on the floor if it seems too hard. Two pillows are needed, one under her head and one under her knees. Her head should fall slightly to one side on the pillow and her arms should lie a few inches from her side, with the elbows half bent outward and the hands half closed. Her knees, supported by a pillow, should be slightly separated, her feet falling outward. It is important to have *all joints in a semiflexed (i.e., slightly bent) position,* for joints as well as muscles must be completely relaxed.

RECOGNIZING TENSION

When we speak of muscle tension, we are referring to tension in the muscles attached to the bones—the skeletal muscles. These are all under the control of the will. With practice they can be tensed or relaxed when so ordered by the mind. While the involuntary muscles of the intestines, blood vessels, heart, lungs, stomach, uterus, etc., cannot be directly relaxed by the will, they are all profoundly influenced by the complete relaxation of the skeletal muscles, which enables them to carry out their respective functions more efficiently.

One cannot be conscious of muscular relaxation unless he is able to recognize muscle tension. This is usually quickly done. I tell my patient to let her arms and legs lie as loosely as she is able to: "Try and avoid moving your toes, and do not wiggle your fingers. Just lie absolutely still and loose on the couch. Now let me have your right arm and let me have it *entirely*. Do not try to help me raise it, because any effort you make to help me is going to do more harm than good."

I then take hold of her elbow and wrist and raise her arm just off the couch. I explain that I want her hand to drop so that there is no "life" in it at all. It is astonishing how many people cannot drop their hand! Because of unnecessary muscle tension they slowly lower their hand, and then wiggle a finger or a thumb.

I continue testing her elbow and wrist until complete relaxation of the hand is obtained. I say again, "Now I am going to lift your hand, and I want you to let it drop absolutely as if it had no life in it at all." This sometimes takes quite a long time to do. Then I put my finger across the back of her hand and say, "Raise your hand very slowly, and at the same time you will feel my finger pressing it down. When you do that, realize what muscles are trying to raise your hand."

At the first movement of the muscles of the forearm in the effort to raise her hand I usually say, "Let it go," or "Relax." We do this several times, and I point out that it is the muscle of the forearm that is trying to raise the hand. Not infrequently my patient observes that as soon as the effort to lift the hand is made, she can feel the muscles tightening.

This instruction is then extended to groups of muscles, allowing them to become slightly tense and then definitely relaxed. It is amazing how quickly the average woman is able to relax her arm, once she understands the muscle tension and the "pull" of the muscle in action, but it takes considerable practice before she becomes expert at releasing this tension. I then ask her to do the same thing with her left arm, and on to other parts of her body.

Instruction is given in a quiet voice, slowly and clearly. "Take a deep breath through an open mouth; curl up your toes and tense the muscles of one leg." Pause. "Release your breath slowly and relax the whole limb. Compare in your own mind the feelings of tension and relaxation." This exercise is repeated, followed by the same procedure with the other leg.

The instruction is then extended to other groups of muscles throughout the body, allowing them to become alternately tense and relaxed, thus discovering what tension of each muscle feels like, and then how it feels to release that tension and relax the muscle. This applies to the chest, back and abdominal muscles as well as the arms and legs. When learning to relax the abdominal muscles, particular attention should also be called to tensing and relaxing the muscles of the pelvic openings, the vaginal and anal passages.

Relaxation of the face is extremely important. A woman who screws up her face in labor is not sufficiently relaxed in other parts of her body. There are about sixty facial muscles that can be tensed, and a woman must be trained to "let go" this tension. It must be remembered that a woman does not look her best when her face is relaxed. I always point this out and tell her that I have no desire for her to look her best, but I want her to *be* her best. I find that the face is probably the most difficult part of the body for a woman to relax.

But women must be taught to release the tension in muscles around their eyes, cheeks, mouth, and especially the eyelids. After a time she who acquires good relaxation of the face finds it very much easier to eliminate tension from her whole body. Any woman who is capable of relaxing her facial muscles at will can go through labor with the maximum ease that the absence of tension makes possible.

As time passes during a period of relaxing, the weight and heaviness of the limbs will be realized. Only with considerable difficulty can one leg be raised slowly from the bed. Recognition of tension versus relaxation will be assisted if the contraction of muscles in the leg is noticed before the heel is raised from the bed. The thigh muscles and those down the front of the leg will produce a distinct sensation of tension if the movements are made sufficiently slowly. The same may be tried with the arm. From the shoulder start to lift the arm— not the hand, but the whole arm—from the bed. The strain upon the muscles will be felt long before there is sufficient force to raise the limb. These tests must be carried out thoughtfully and *very slowly*. Violent and sudden flinging of the arm or the leg into the air will undoubtedly be easy, but it will teach nothing of the sensations of relaxation and early tension. Having raised the limb one or two inches from the bed, let it fall. In this way a consciousness of muscle tension will be developed, which makes the practice of deep relaxation much easier to recognize and practice.

When a person becomes physically relaxed, the mind takes care of itself. Several patients have told me that it is very difficult for their imaginations to become quiet. All the events of the day are vividly recalled as soon as they try to relax. This is, of course, an indication that their relaxation is incomplete. But they should not be urged to avoid thought in any way, because the attempt to stop thought is one of the most *active* mental exercises! Instead, it must be remembered that no emotional state can be present if there is real relaxation of the muscles of the body. Thought is to be concentrated on relaxing these muscles. As the muscles relax, the mind itself will automatically become quieter, until thoughts fade.

PRACTICING RELAXATION

It is not necessary to tense the muscles of the body each time in order to relax, once one has learned to recognize the *difference* between tension and relaxation in any part of the body. For each practice session, the following procedure may be carried out:

1. The bladder should first be emptied, so that the pelvic muscles can be relaxed with safety. Then stand and stretch the whole body, breathing in deeply through the nose to full lung capacity. Then exhale, allowing the shoulders to drop and the head to fall forward as the lungs become empty.

2. Lie down on a wide couch, the floor, or a hard bed, with a pillow under your head *and the upper part of your shoulders* (fig. 22). Another pillow should be made into a roll and placed under your knees for support, so that both knee and hip joints are slightly bent.

3. The feet should be about six or eight inches apart. Arms should be eight inches to a foot away from the body, with the elbows flexed outward, the hands with palms down and fingers curled slightly inward. The head should be allowed to fall gently to one side on the pillow, with the chin slightly raised as the head falls back.

4. Take three or four slow deep breaths and, on breathing out each time, let every muscle in the body become limp and still. Think of the shoulders as "opening outward." Feel the arms hanging from the shoulders and the hands lying heavily on the bed. Fingers and thumbs must not move. There will be a sensation of sinking into, or even through, the bed. The feet fall outward upon the heels, and the knees are carried outward by the weight of the feet (fig. 23). There must be no movement of the toes.

5. The head and shoulders are to be so completely sup-

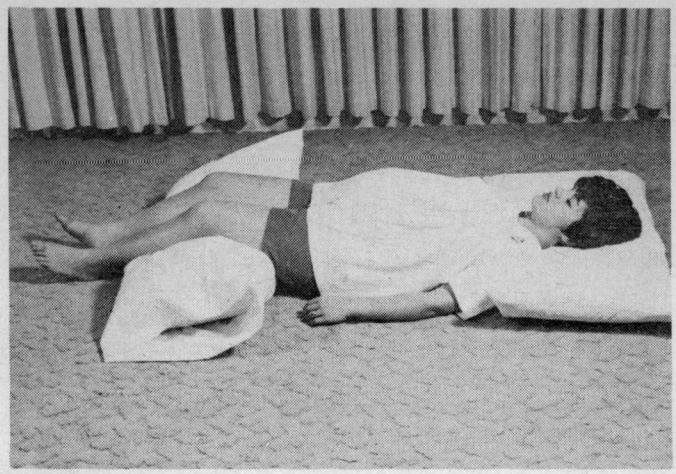

Fig. 22. Relaxation on back in earlier pregnancy. Pillow under head should be down under neck and shoulders, as shown here.

Fig. 23. Note the excellent relaxation of legs and feet, knees falling outward, feet inward. Head is incorrectly supported, neck bent forward because the pillow does not come down under neck and shoulders as in Fig. 22.

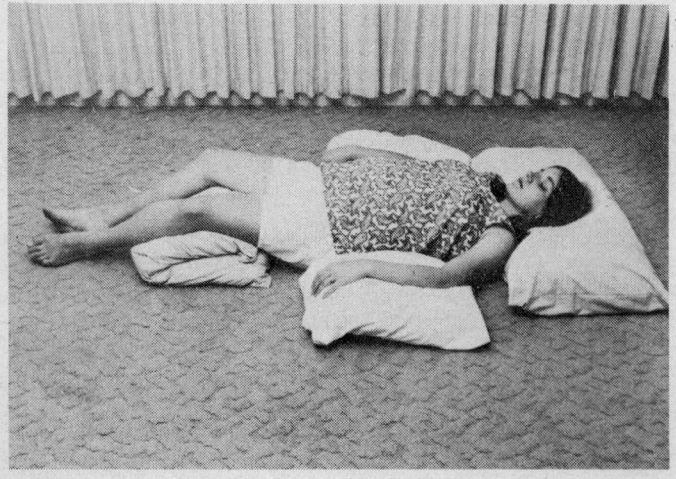

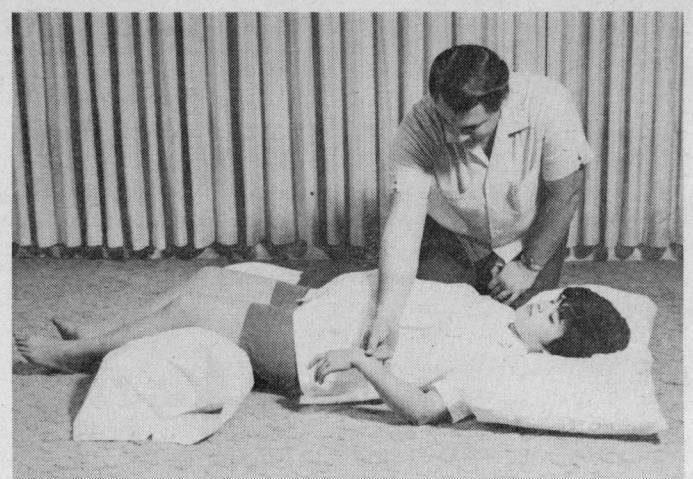

Fig. 24. Husband checking limpness of arm muscles, flexibility of elbow, wrist, and finger joints.

Fig. 25. Husband checking limpness of thigh and leg, flexibility of hip, knee, and ankle joints.

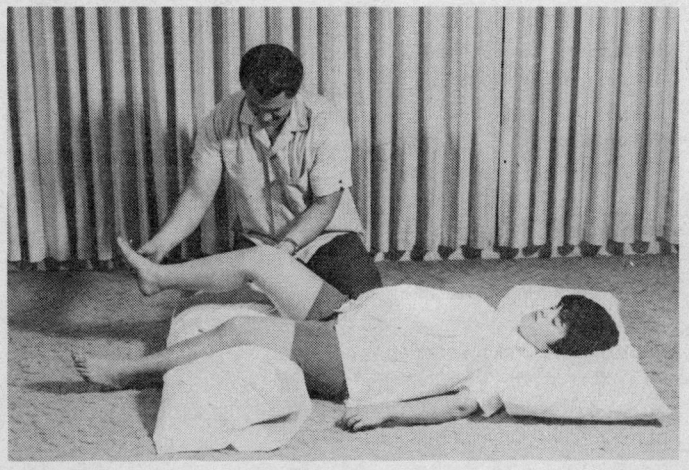

ported upon the pillow that the muscles of the neck are absolutely loose. Let the eyelids half close of their own weight.

6. Concentrate briefly on each arm without moving or tensing it, to be sure it is not being held stiffly in any part, that the muscles are not twitching or the fingers fidgeting (fig. 24). Do the same with the legs, buttocks, and back. Note carefully the muscles of the back. If they are relaxed, there will be a sensation of pressure upon the bed or floor from the weight of your body.

7. Relax the muscles of the face, the brow, eyelids, cheeks, and the muscles around the mouth. Think of your head as making a dent in the pillow. Particular care must be taken not to blink the eyes or move the eyeballs within their sockets. The muscles of the face will be felt hanging loosely from the cheekbones, which causes the jaw to drop slightly and hang loose.

8. Release any remaining tension in the abdominal muscles and pelvic floor muscles. Take two or three breaths deeply into the diaphragm, letting the chest and abdominal wall collapse with its own weight slowly as each breath is exhaled. Allow the breath to leave the lungs through the mouth without controlling or impeding it. Do not force it out. After each expiration, pause for two seconds (or until you want a new breath) before inhaling into the diaphragm again, deeply and gently. With each outgoing breath, relax the abdominal wall more fully, and "let go" tension in the pelvic muscles, as if opening up down below. Remember to keep your lips parted and your cheeks and jaw "hanging loose," to help relax the pelvic area. If your mouth is tense, you will be tensing the pelvic area, too. As relaxation deepens, the "sleep" breathing will become very gentle and quiet, as if you were really asleep. It is not necessary to remain conscious of the breathing pattern once full relaxation is achieved.

9. Let all the joints of the body relax a little more with each outgoing breath until they seem to be detached altogether (fig.

25). Note the train of sensations in the limbs—usually heaviness followed by lightness or "floating"; faint, transient pins and needles in the hands; feelings of warmth passing up from the extremities.

10. A pleasant, daydreaming state generally ensues (as in sunbathing) and any tendency to directed thinking should be deliberately diverted into a daydream. Remain in this relaxed state for about half an hour. (The sense of the passage of time is often lost or blunted.) Sleep is not the aim, and for most patients muscular relaxation without falling asleep seems to be more refreshing. But relaxing again in this way at night will help many insomniacs put themselves to sleep.

11. *Get up slowly*. Jumping up suddenly may cause faintness or dizziness. Take two or three deep breaths, bend the knees and arms once or twice, and then slowly sit up. Take two or three more breaths before standing up. Stretch the body once more, and then normal movement may again be safely resumed.

BREATHING

Breathing can be demonstrated to be either tense or relaxed. If too deep a breath is forced, or breathing is too rapid, certain tensions become apparent in the diaphragm, the ribs, and elsewhere. In relaxed breathing, both breathing in and breathing out should be without tension. "Sleep" breathing— that is, drawing the air into the lower diaphragm rather than the upper chest—aids in achieving relaxation more quickly and deeply. As the person relaxes, the abdominal wall will gently rise and fall. But as relaxation becomes deeper, breathing becomes perfectly smooth and in many cases almost inaudible, for less oxygen is needed during relaxation than when in a state of tension or movement. This quiet breathing is quite adequate to carry on all respiratory functions in labor during the first stage, without any necessity for shortness of breath, panting, or occasional deep breaths or sighs. All these breathing variations are signs of tension and incomplete relaxation, which will cause the contractions to become uncomfortable.

POSITIONS FOR RELAXATION

1. *On the back.* This position has been described above. However, after eighteen to twenty weeks of pregnancy many women have difficulty being comfortable in this position.

2. *Reclining chair position.* The body rests at an angle of 45 to 50 degrees, the forearms relaxing on the arms of the chair and the knees relaxing on the lower portion of the chair, tilted slightly higher than the hips. The head should be supported and fall slightly to one side, so that the neck muscles are slack and no part of the body requires any muscular effort to remain in its position.

In the hospital, this same position can be attained by raising the head of the bed to the proper angle, and either placing pillows under the knees to elevate them, or raising the bed under the knees, if it has that kind of mechanical flexibility (fig. 26). Pillows should be placed under the elbows to simulate the arms of a chair, and the head and shoulders should be so well supported that the neck muscles are fully relaxed, with the head falling slightly to the side and backward.

3. *Lateral position.* This is a most important position, and should be learned as an alternative to the other positions in early pregnancy, even though it may not be necessary at that time. In the later months, when the uterus is large, it is usually uncomfortable to lie flat on the back, for this interferes with good circulation and, because of the pressure of the uterus within the abdomen, makes breathing difficult. The lateral position is most helpful during labor.

Lie on the bed or floor on the left side, with the left arm behind the back and lying relaxed alongside the body. The right shoulder should be dropped, or supported by a corner of the pillow, and the right arm flexed slightly at the elbow and resting loosely on the bed alongside the pillow (fig. 27). It is important to either support the right shoulder or make sure it drops forward, as there is a tendency for muscle tension to hold it up. The head should be resting on a pillow, face turned toward the right shoulder, the chin slightly raised to make breathing easier, lips parted, and jaw slack.

The left leg should be stretched out on the bed, but bent slightly at the knee to relax the knee and hip joints, and the right leg should be drawn up until the knee is on a level with the upper abdomen. A large, firm pillow should be placed under the right knee and thigh to give it support, so that the knee and hip joints are fully relaxed and loose, and the muscles of the upper thigh, abdomen, lower back, and pelvic area can hang completely slack (fig. 28).

Two or three deep breaths into the lower diaphragm should be taken, and the whole body made to "let go" more fully with each exhalation. A sense of comfort and support will be felt immediately, if the position is right (fig. 29). The uterus will be supported upon the bed without pressure, taking the strain off the back muscles. Free movement of the diaphragm and abdomen is obtained during breathing.

During early pregnancy this position may also be used while lying on the right side. Relaxation is equally effective while lying on either side, but in later pregnancy, and when in early labor, the *left* lateral position is the best position (figs. 30, 31).

RESIDUAL TENSION

The difference between simply lying still and true neuromuscular relaxation can be recognized, by a competent observer, in indications of residual tension. A rapid pulse rate and certain nervous reactions and reflexes are the result of tension. But the physician can also diagnose tension by listening to the breathing of a woman, for any irregularity in her breathing is evidence of imperfect relaxation. The flicker of an

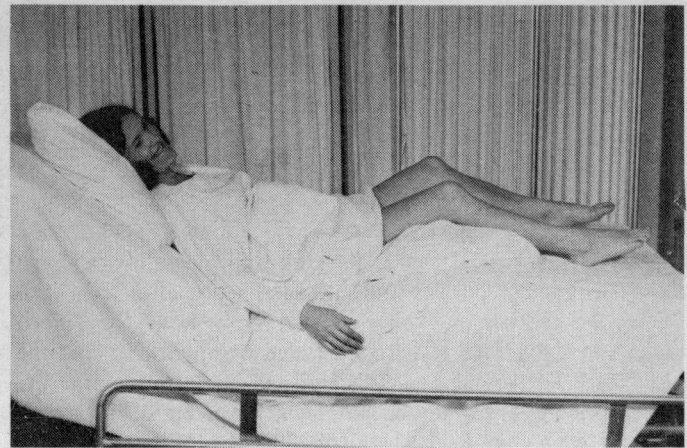

Fig. 26. "Reclining chair" position for relaxation in labor. Pillows under the forearms (not shown) may be helpful in keeping arms limp.

Fig. 27. Left lateral relaxation. Lie on left side, left arm and shoulder resting on floor, arm bent at the elbow. The corner of the pillow on which the head rests is to be brought down under the right shoulder and forearm also, so that they are fully supported by the pillow, and completely relaxed. The right forearm rests on the floor, not on the pillow.

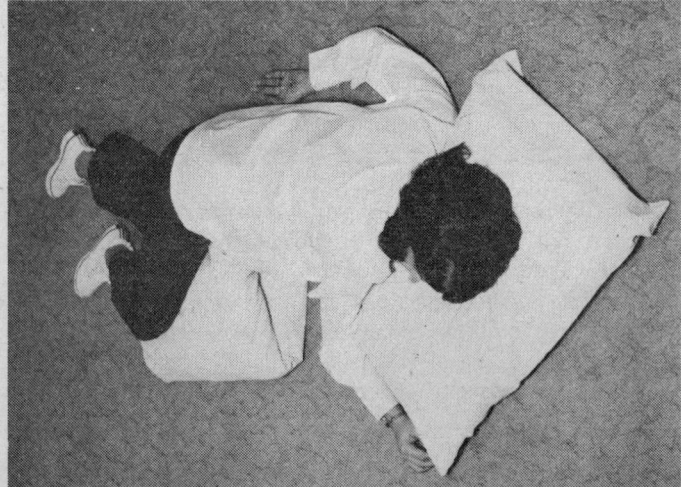

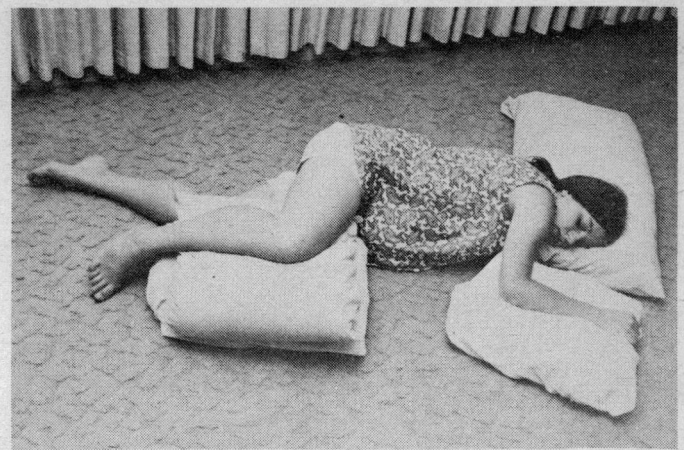

Fig. 28. Left lateral relaxation. Lie on left side, left leg bent at the knee and resting on the floor. Bend the right knee and draw it up toward the body, placing a pillow under it. The right upper thigh and knee must be *fully supported* by an ample pillow, so that all the leg and back muscles are completely relaxed (slack).

Fig. 29. Husband learning to check relaxation during a contraction.

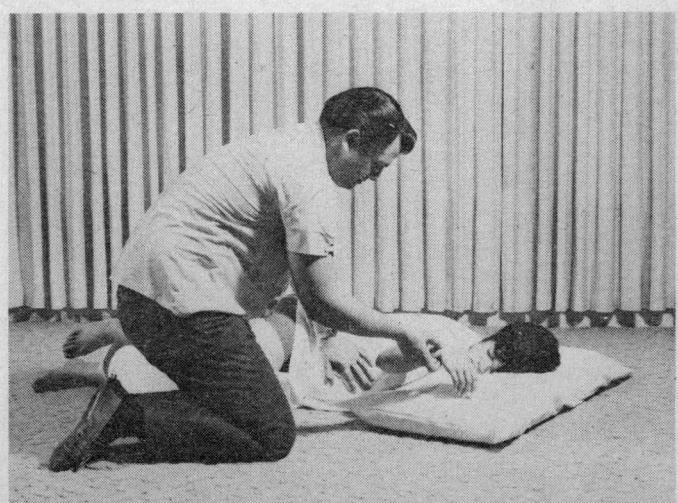

Fig. 30. Practicing relaxation in left lateral position during pregnancy.

Fig. 31. Relaxing in left lateral position during first-stage labor.

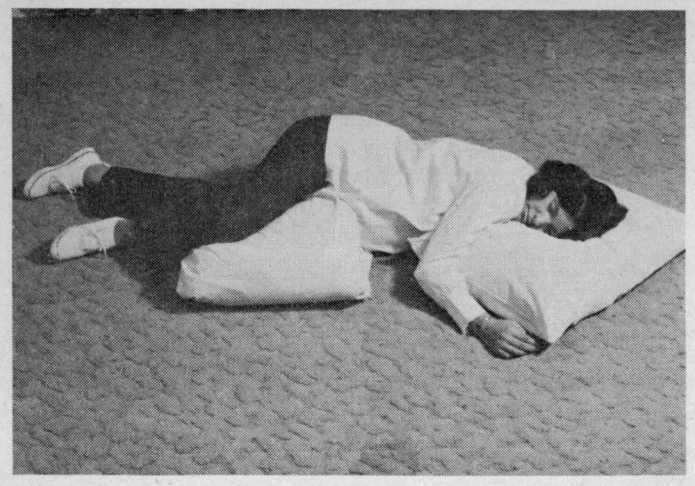

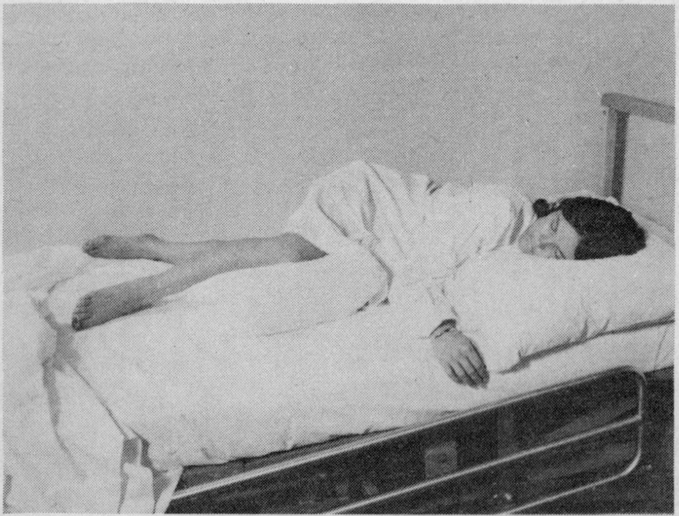

eyelid, moving of her eyeballs in their sockets behind closed lids, shifting of a finger or toe, or swallowing, all demonstrate the presence of residual tension of which the woman herself is not aware. If, in the silence of a relaxing class the instructress makes a sudden slight noise, she will notice those who react immediately to this disturbance.

The aim should be to train women to relax until all residual tension is eliminated, but at the same time realize that the instruction received at prenatal classes alone is not enough to achieve this desirable state in every woman. Those who do overcome residual tension are usually the perfect obstetric patients, providing they have no disproportion and the baby is lying in the normal position. But every woman benefits by the measure of relaxation she learns, for any lessening of tension in labor lessens discomfort by just that much. The experienced obstetrician will realize that no one can prophesy with certainty the conduct of any woman in labor, although it is possible to detect those who appear likely to do well, and to predict those who are more likely to find relaxing difficult.

Perhaps I may add that the obstetrician himself would be very well advised to become adept at relaxation. Not only would he be more competent to teach his patients or train instructresses, but he would find himself retaining his energy during those long hours of waiting. His mental acuity and manual dexterity would be more efficient also, than if he had remained tense with anticipation during his attendance at the labor.

5

Physical Fitness

There is no reason why a woman has to become fat and ungainly in order to become a mother; indeed, there is no reason why she should not have an even better figure after she has borne a child than before, for the benefits derived from exercises are the same whether a woman is pregnant or not. When exercises are undertaken seriously, the physical condition rapidly improves and a sense of well-being takes the place of the lethargy so frequently found among people whose lives do not include enough physical activity.

Certain movements associated with the mobility and flexibility of the muscles and joints of the pelvis are valuable during labor and delivery. Others assist in the depth and control of breathing. When we visualize the course of normal labor, we realize that the first stage must be without muscular effort on the part of the woman, while the second stage may require an hour or two of physical effort, in the case of first labors, to help the uterus expel the infant.

But we must not exaggerate the importance of exercises for childbirth. They make the mother feel fit and help correct breathing and relaxation, but a woman with a well-trained mind who knows how to breathe and relax correctly, but is unable for some health reason to do any exercises, can still have a good birth experience. She will have her baby much more easily than will a woman who has a highly trained athletic body but who knows little or nothing of how to cooperate with nature in giving birth. Indeed, some of the most perfect labors I have witnessed have been of women with groups of muscles partially paralyzed below the waist. They had suffered from accidents or polio, and their crippled bodies, which they swung from the hips on crutches or walking sticks, could not be physically trained.

I am anxious that this be understood, for the exercises described in this chapter are not to prepare mothers for an athletic event, but for a natural, common-sense experience in which a certain degree of physical fitness has advantages. These exercises represent the most elementary practice of physical training, but they are enough. Anything more than sufficient has been shown by experience to make *no difference* to the course or comfort of labor. Anything less deprives a woman of advantages she might more easily have enjoyed by being in better health.

POSTURE

Correct posture enables a woman to move gracefully and to breathe freely. A straight line from the ear to a point just in front of the heel on the sole of the foot should pass through the center of the shoulder and the hip joint, enabling the muscles of the limbs to work to the best advantage in all directions and retaining the abdominal organs in good position within the pelvic cavity. Holding the head at such an angle avoids round shoulders and the poking forward of the chin, and holding the body in this position makes breathing free, deep, and effortless and gives one a feeling of well-being and cheerfulness, which is important.

A woman can adopt the correct position by standing near a mirror and picturing the imaginary line just described. Her head should be carried as though slightly above her height. She should check her posture in this way periodically through pregnancy, for the alteration in the shape and weight of the body during pregnancy will unconsciously lead to stooping unless attention is paid to it. There is nothing more attractive than a young pregnant woman moving freely and maintaining her personal appearance in good posture.

EXERCISES

The following exercises are to be done slowly, remaining deliberately aware of each movement. Breathing and muscular action are to be coordinated in an easy rhythm without holding the breath, except in one exercise. All the exercises are simple, and no strain is required to do them satisfactorily. No exercises are done with the arms above the head. Shoulder height is the maximum to which the arms should be raised in any prenatal exercises.

Exercise 1: Pelvic Rock

This loosens and mobilizes the lower spine and pelvic joints. It prevents and sometimes relieves backache.

On hands and knees, place the hands about twelve inches apart and the knees about nine inches apart, keeping the knees directly in line with the hips. Let the back sag, at the same time raising the buttocks as high as possible (fig. 32). Take a deep breath in this position.

Slowly raise the back, allowing the breath to be expelled as the back arches (fig. 33). At the same time, squeeze together the muscles of the buttocks and pelvic area and tighten the muscles of the upper legs.

Return to the original position and *repeat ten times,* slowly and firmly.

Exercise 2: Squatting (with Variations)

These exercises loosen the knees and the hip joints, tone up the muscles of the legs, and stretch the muscles on the inside of the thighs. This exercise parallels the best position for delivery of the child, for in the squatting position the pelvic diameter is enlarged to its maximum size.

Stand on the toes, and then sink down to a position of squatting or sitting on the heels, still balancing on the toes. Place the palms of the hands on the knees and stretch the legs wide open, keeping the back straight (fig. 34). Rise to a standing position and then lower the heels to the floor. If the balance cannot be maintained, hold on to a support with one hand. *Repeat five times.*

VARIATION (a). For those who find the squatting too difficult or too strenuous, the same exercise can be simulated while lying on the back, with the knees drawn up toward the chest and pressed together (fig. 35). Allow the knees to fall outward, pressing them widely apart with the palms of the hands, the soles of the feet pointing inward (fig. 36). *Repeat five times.*

VARIATION (b). Sit on the floor Indian style, with knees outward, the soles of the feet placed together. Grasp the ankles with each hand, lean forward and place the forearms on the lower legs, then gently press the knees apart with the elbows (fig. 37). *Repeat five times.*

VARIATION (c). Sitting Indian style as in variation b, grasp the ankles but keep the arms straight. Let your husband or an attendant push down against the knees while you try to *push* up against the pressure of his hands (fig. 38). (Important note to husbands: Do not force too hard! Crunching her knees to the floor may cause damage.) *Repeat five times.*

VARIATION (d). Sit Indian style (fig. 39), crossing ankles, often during the day for quiet work, reading, sewing, or watching TV. Try relaxing occasionally in this position, letting the elbows rest on the knees, the back sag, and the head drop gently forward, eyes closed.

Exercise 3: Firming the Breasts

This exercise increases the circulation to the tissues under the breasts, strengthens the muscles supporting the breasts,

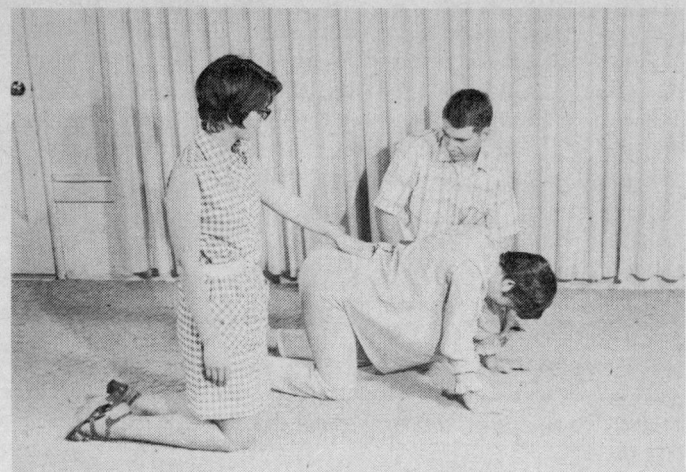

Fig. 32. Pelvic rocking. Let back sag, keeping elbows straight, knees directly under hips.

Fig. 33. Slowly raise small of back as far as possible, keeping legs from knees up at right angles to the floor.

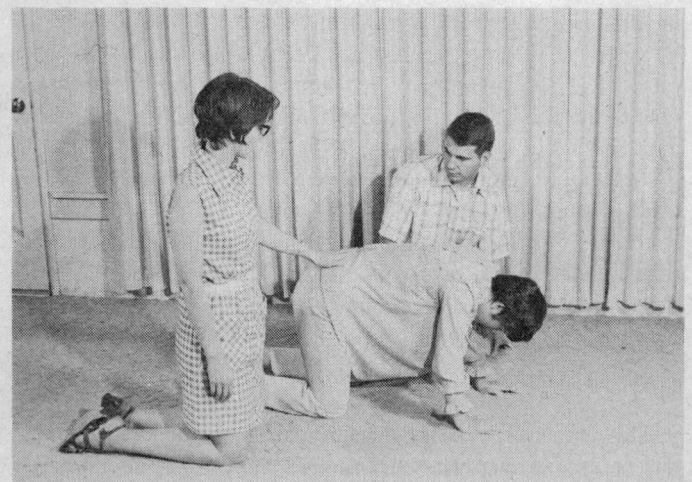

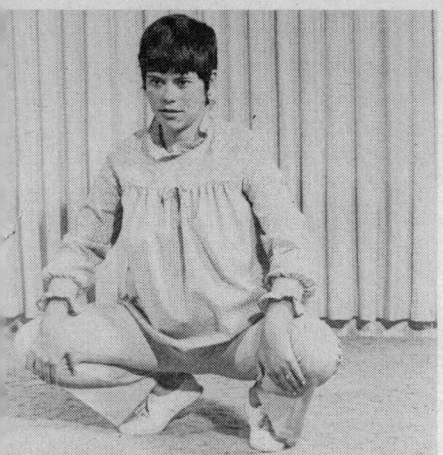

Fig. 34. Squat, balancing on toes. Press knees open with hands.

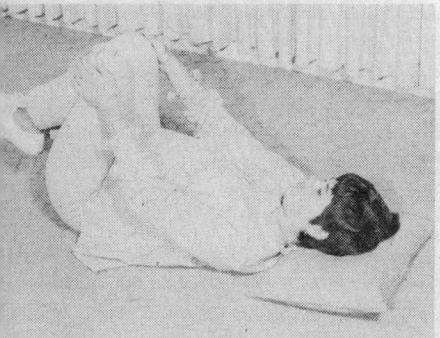

Fig. 35. Draw knees up toward chest, press together with hands.

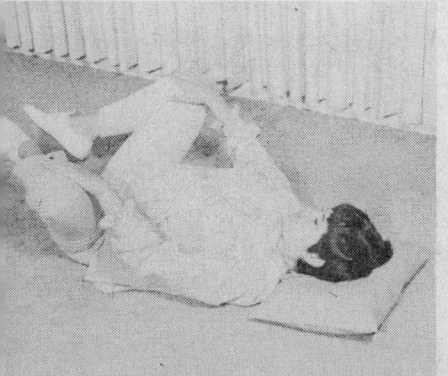

Fig. 36. Press knees as far apart as possible with palms of hands.

Fig. 37. Soles of feet together, press knees apart with elbows, grasping ankles.

Fig. 38. Soles of feet together, push knees up against husband's hands.

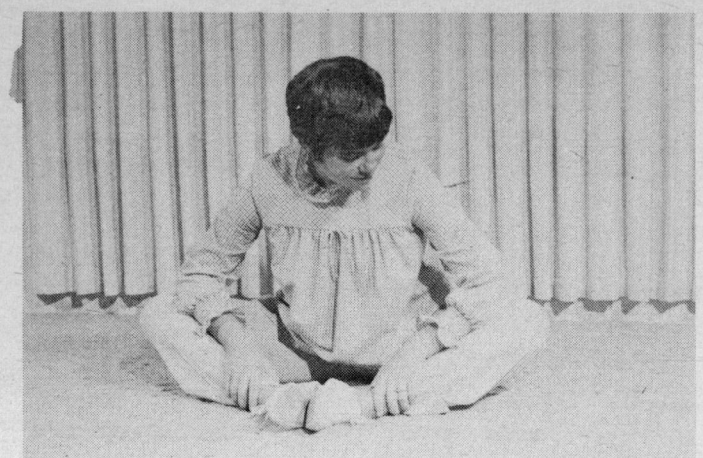

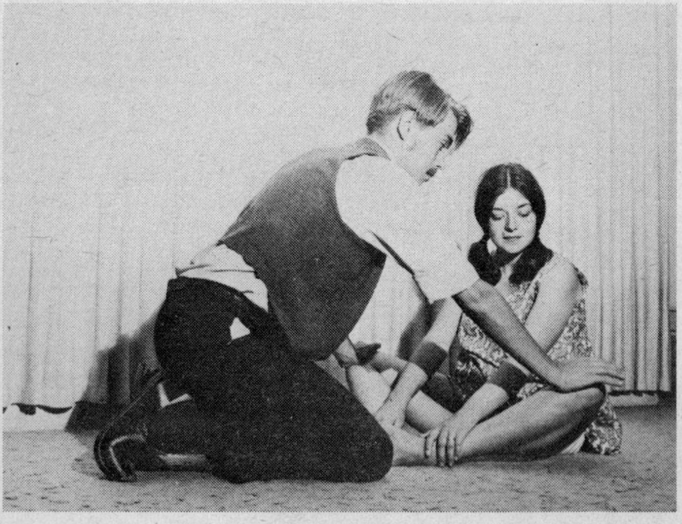

and also seems to help in establishing an adequate milk flow for breastfeeding. This is the only exercise that also gives practice in holding the breath.

Grip each arm firmly behind the wrist and raise the arms to the level of the shoulders. Push the skin of the forearm up, tightening the arm muscles and the muscles of the chest (fig. 40). When done correctly, one can feel the breasts lift. Relax and repeat.

Now take a deep breath, and hold it while doing this exercise *ten times,* taking about ten seconds. Relax. This time is to be gradually increased until the breath can be held comfortably for twenty seconds, which is a considerable help in the expulsive stage of labor, while the mother pushes, before she can exhale.

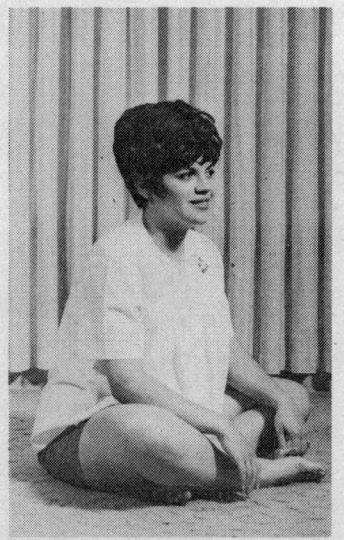

Fig. 39. Sitting Indian style.

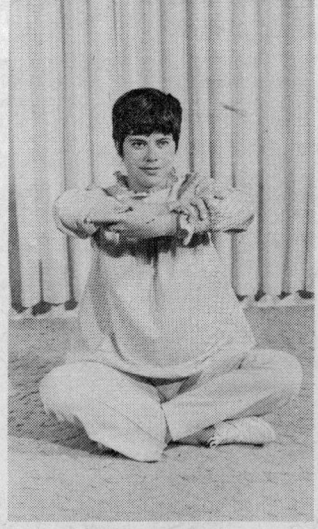

Fig. 40. Exercise for lifting and firming the breasts.

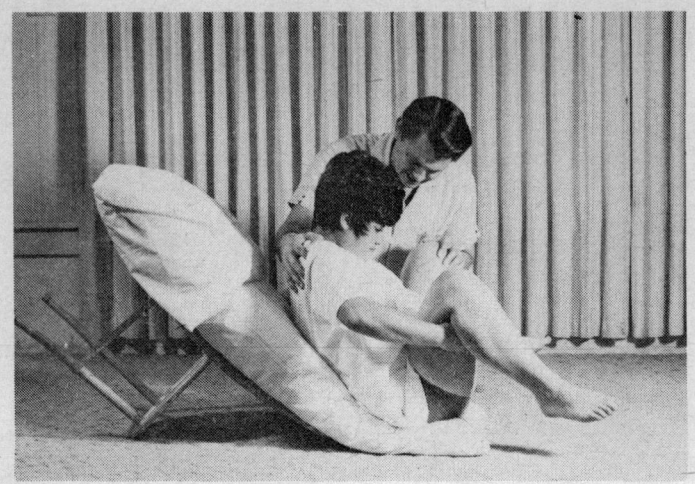

Fig. 41. Practice position for bearing down.

Fig. 42. Bearing down with contractions in second-stage labor.

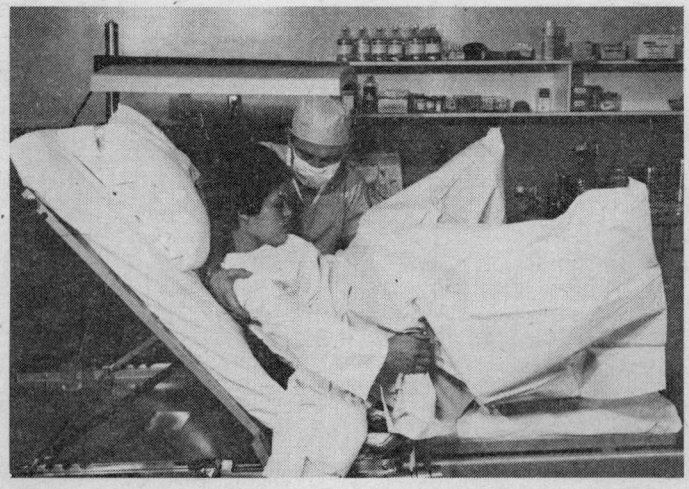

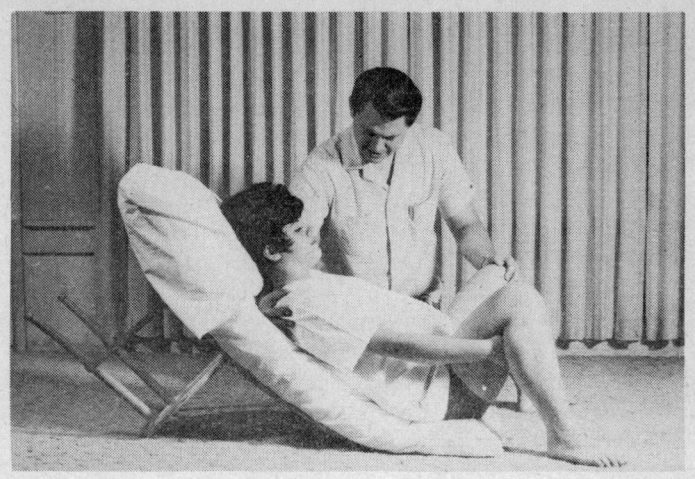

Fig. 43. Practice rest position in second-stage labor.

Fig. 44. Relaxed and happy between pushing with second-stage contractions.

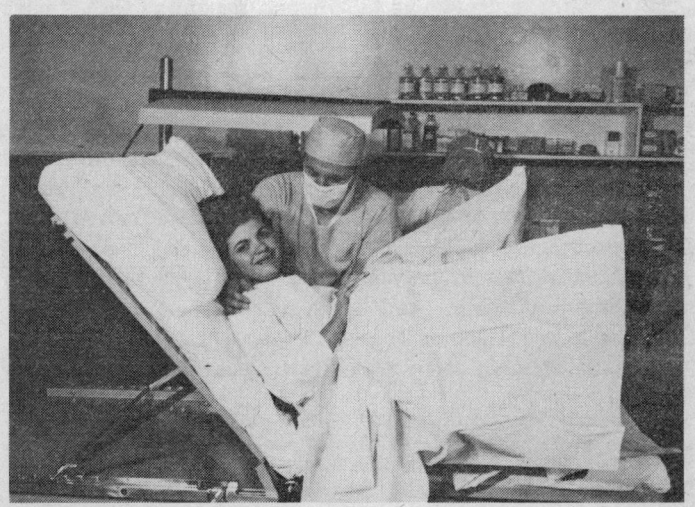

Exercise 4: Labor ("Work") Position

During the last two months of pregnancy this position should be practiced, as it is the most comfortable and advantageous while giving birth.

Rest with the back on an inverted chair padded with pillows at an angle of 40 to 45 degrees to the bed or floor. Draw the knees up to the sides of the abdomen toward the shoulders, grasp under each knee with the hands, bend the head forward and pull the knees up and *as widely apart as possible* (figs. 41, 42, 43, 44). When the knees are at their widest, the soles of the feet will be turned partially inward toward each other.

Exercise 5: Firming the Pelvic Floor Muscles*

This is the most important of all prenatal and postnatal exercises, and requires some explanation in detail.

The anus, vagina, and urethra are the three openings in the female pelvis. The anus is the end of the bowel; the vagina, the end of the birth canal; and the urethra, the end of the urinary bladder. When standing, the force of gravity places an immense strain upon the muscles that support the floor of the pelvis and close the openings.

Contract the anal and vaginal passages firmly and at the same time tighten the buttocks. Close the anus until the sensation of drawing it up into the rectum is felt. There is no need to move the legs or buttocks, as this distracts attention from the important area. When the anal sphincter is completely closed and retracted, the vaginal sphincter, the *levator ani*—a large internal muscle—and the sphincter of the urine outlet are also tensed. Each of these openings is surrounded by fibers of muscle arranged as a double figure eight; therefore all three

---

* Arnold Kegel, M.D., gynecologist at the University of Southern California, has perfected and promoted pubococcygeal exercises in the United States so extensively that they are often simply called "the Kegel."

outlets are closed by what is virtually one muscle. Squeeze these muscles as tightly as possible, hold for a definite pause, and relax *slowly*. By relaxing slowly, one learns how to "let go" tension in these muscles. Do this exercise at least *twelve times, twice a day*. It can be done any time, anywhere. As the uterus grows, the blood vessels multiply in number and increase in size. If the tone of the outlet muscles is below normal standard, control over them is lessened. Urine may leak, particularly during laughing or coughing. Similar defects may arise in the anus, as well as the development of *hemorrhoids,* or *piles*—varicose veins of the anus. If the muscles of the pelvic floor and outlets are exercised and kept in tone, these troubles will occur less frequently.

This exercise also facilitates the restoring of the stretched and dilated openings to normal size and tone after labor, and prevents some of the minor discomforts of aging. The feeling of firmness underneath has a marked influence on a woman; she will move or stand in a more confident posture.

Controlled activity of the vaginal sphincter and the static tension of the pelvic floor are also assets of considerable domestic value. Coitus can be performed satisfactorily for both husband and wife when the wife has learned conscious control of the vaginal sphincter. Rather than the too-frequent complaint that intercourse is uninteresting after a woman has had a baby, I am told from time to time that this natural marital function is performed more satisfactorily than before.

This simple exercise is a panacea for many ills and should be taught to and performed habitually by all women—whether pregnant, postparturient, or just woman!

6

Labor: First-Stage Labor

Two hundred and eighty days is an arbitrary figure for the length of pregnancy, calculated from the first day of the last menstrual period. (The average actual length from conception to birth is estimated as 267 days.) But a baby may be full term and quite normal if it arrives at any time between 265 and 290 days. It must not be thought, therefore, that a baby born ten days before the expected date is necessarily premature, or ten days after is postmature. A woman under my care had all three of her children on the three-hundredth day from the first day of her last menstrual period. She had very easy labors, and there was no evidence that any of the children were overdue. When a baby is "ripe" and ready, labor will begin.

ONSET OF LABOR

There are three signs that labor is beginning:

1. *Rhythmical contractions of the uterus.* These are felt as sensations of tightness without discomfort in the abdomen. The uterus becomes hard and tightness can be felt all over the organ. The importance of the sign is in the *rhythm* and not the contractions. A pregnant woman may have definite contractions for some weeks before her baby is due, but, if a regular and continuous rhythm is not established, they do not usually indicate the onset of labor. True labor contractions may start once every ten or fifteen minutes, or even at longer intervals, but gradually the interval decreases until they come every

three or four minutes. There is no pain as long as the abdomen is relaxed.

2. *Leaking of the waters.* The bag of waters may leak slowly, or it may suddenly burst and the waters flow out in a gush. This occasionally occurs before the uterus starts its rhythmical contractions, but this is true more frequently with subsequent babies than with the first. There is no pain when the bag of waters bursts, though it may be startling. It is wise to notify a doctor immediately. Rhythmical contractions may begin in an hour or two if they have not begun previously, or they may not begin for two or three days. But it is an indication that labor will soon be under way, so the woman should be under her doctor's advisement.

3. *The show.* A slight discharge of blood and mucus, known as "the show," may appear. It usually occurs after uterine contractions have begun to dilate the cervix slightly, thus dislodging the plug of mucus that kept the cervix sealed during pregnancy. This is positive evidence of the onset of labor.

Any one of these three major signs usually makes it easy for a woman to realize that her baby is on the way. She should get in touch with her doctor, even if there is some doubt in her mind, and follow his advice on when to leave for the hospital.

EARLY FIRST-STAGE LABOR

Once labor has begun and the doctor been notified, "plenty of time" should be the motto, with no hurry or anxiety unless the hospital is a long distance away. Small chores can be attended to around the house in preparation for leaving. Often there is excitement and relief that the day has come, which gives rise to a flurry of last-minute activity. This distraction helps the uterus settle down to its work without too much attention until labor is steadily under way. The doctor will advise when to go to the hospital, probably not, for a first baby, before contractions are five to ten minutes apart.

Upon arrival at the hospital (figs. 45, 46) the mother is

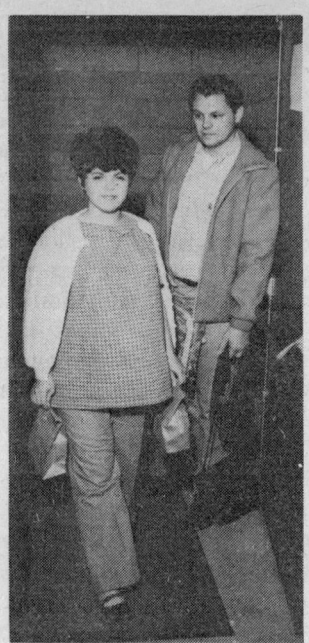

Fig. 45. Arrival at hospital in labor.

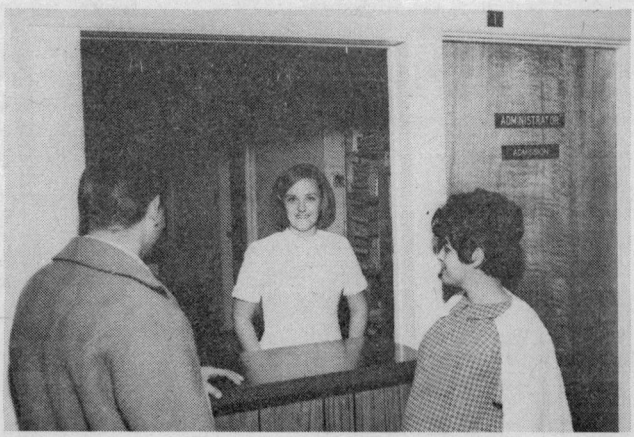

Fig. 46. Being greeted by receptionist.

greeted by a receptionist and taken immediately to a labor room if labor is progressing rapidly. If not, she is identified by her prenatal records and admitted according to the usual obstetric routine. She is weighed, her blood pressure taken, and a specimen of urine examined.

Once in the labor room she is prepared for an examination by her doctor or a medical attendant. This preparation must be in keeping with the written instructions of her own physician. No enema, perineal shaving, analgesics, amnesics, sedatives, fluids or oxytocics are to be given except on his written orders specifically for her.* During the medical examination the physician will determine how far along she is in labor, listen to the baby's heart, and determine its position by examination of the abdomen.

I do not advise that during the first stage of the average labor a woman should be asked to relax the whole time unless she wishes it, unless she has overcome all the difficulties of progressive relaxation and is adept at the art. In the ordinary labor I prefer the woman to be awake to her general condition, able to listen to instruction and learn what is going on, and able to recognize the encouragement given her by those in attendance. But as soon as there is a sign of a uterine contraction, she must at once apply herself and relax to the very best of her ability.

A quiet restfulness between contractions is sufficient. Many women read or sew duing the earlier part of the first stage (fig. 47). Some prefer to walk about, if the waters have not yet broken. Undisturbed peace should characterize the first stage of labor—without mental or physical tension, with every happiness that a woman can be given, and with every encouragement to be confident in the right outcome of her labor.

Sometimes, when labor is slow in making progress, a mild sedative may be beneficial to help her rest peacefully or sleep.

* See *Standards for Obstetric-Gynecologic Hospital Services* (Chicago: The American College of Obstetricians and Gynecologists, 1969).

A few hours' sleep, particularly at night, during the early dilatation of the cervix evades the weariness of mind and body that causes a woman to begin to interpret any sensation as painful. This therapeutic common sense should not be confused with the use of drugs to relieve pain. No woman should have to go without sleep for fifteen or twenty hours of a slow first stage.

Adequate nourishment through liquids is also important during the first stage of labor, to sustain her energy and avoid fatigue. Milk, orange juice, tea, and other liquids should be given in ample amounts. During this same period of waiting, the husband should be given full meals at every mealtime, without his leaving her bedside (fig. 48).

When the first stage of labor is well established, a woman should be in a room with a nurse or physician in constant attendance. The companionship of her husband is also invaluable at this time, particularly if he has been trained in helping her remain relaxed and comfortable (fig. 49).

As rhythmical contractions of the uterus increase in intensity, gradually dilating the cervix, there is a demand for patience. If the training that has been given in deep, quiet breathing and complete relaxation is well and truly carried out during contractions, this period of waiting is much less taxing on a woman's patience. The routine of becoming *completely flaccid*, especially in the abdominal and pelvic area during a contraction, will help her improve her skill as time goes on.

When the opening of the cervix is about two inches, or five centimeters, in diameter, most women will begin to feel the strain of waiting, becoming impatient with contractions that seem to be doing no good. They may become restless, not relax as well during contractions as before, and thus begin to have some discomfort. A nurse or medical assistant should recognize that this is a typical emotional reaction, and make every effort to reassure the patient by explaining what is happening, and coach her carefully in reestablishing adequate relaxation and controlled deep breathing with each contraction, until she is comfortable once more.

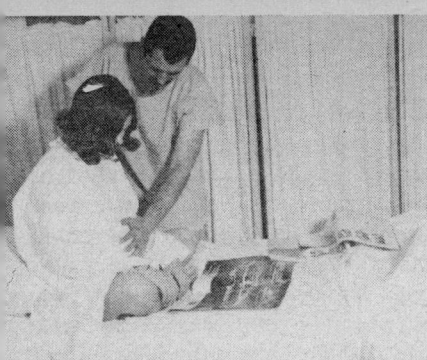

Fig. 47. Quiet activity during early first-stage labor.

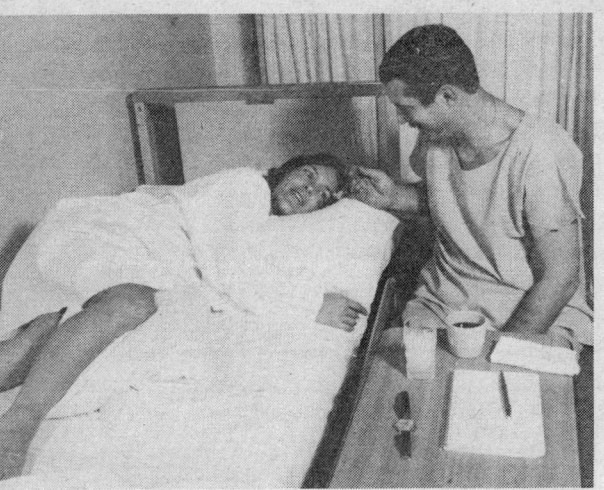

Fig. 48. Husband in constant attendance. Notice his watch, pen, and paper for timing contractions; his coffee (or meals); liquid for the wife.

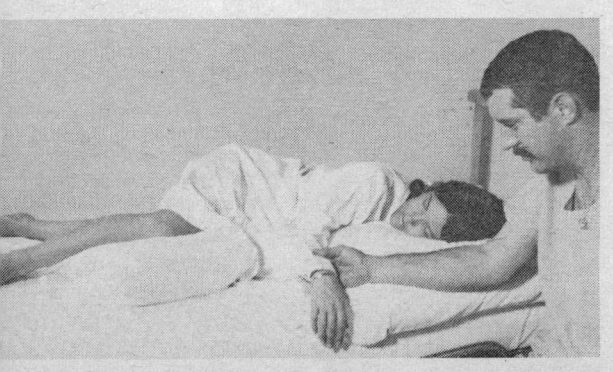

Fig. 49. Complete muscular relaxation during contractions of first stage.

At this time the woman should lay aside any other work such as reading or sewing and assume the labor position most comfortable for her (either the "reclining chair" or the left lateral* position). She should remain fairly relaxed between contractions in order to deepen the level of relaxation *during* each one. Her husband will be a most beneficial influence in helping her become comfortable, as they begin to practice together in earnest what they have learned she is to do during labor (figs. 50, 51, 52, 53). Thus as the contractions become stronger and closer together her ability to relax improves and discomfort fades. But even though she has overcome this first period of anxiety and is relaxing well, she still *must not be left alone*.

LATE FIRST-STAGE LABOR

Position

As labor progresses and the contractions come more quickly and become stronger, the woman should assume the left lateral position for relaxation, as described earlier. It is important that the patient lie in the *left* lateral position, and that she never lie flat on her back during labor, or during late pregnancy. The supine position interferes with adequate circulation.† Before assuming this position, she should make certain that her bladder is empty. All her joints must be loose and bent slightly, her knee and upper thigh firmly supported by a large, firm pillow. She must consciously "let go" all muscular tension in the upper thigh, lower abdomen, and

---

* "Angiographic studies have visualized occlusion of the vena cava, as well as displacement and partial obstruction of the aorta, almost consistently in the supine position during late pregnancy." From J. Bieniarz, *et al.*, "Aortocaval Compression by the Uterus in Late Human Pregnancy. IV. Circulatory Homeostasis by Preferential Perfusion of the Placenta," *American Journal of Obstetrics and Gynecology* 103 (1969): 19–31. Reprinted by permission.

† See *American Journal of Obstetrics and Gynecology* 103: 19–31; *op. cit.*

IN LABOR FOR TWINS

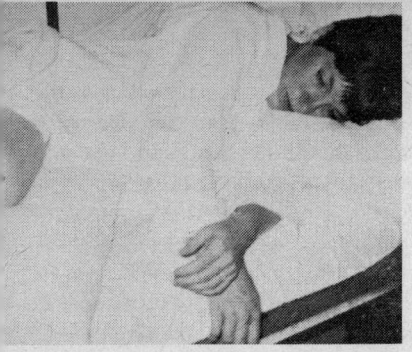

Fig. 50. Relaxing on left side rather than left lateral. Pillow between knees.

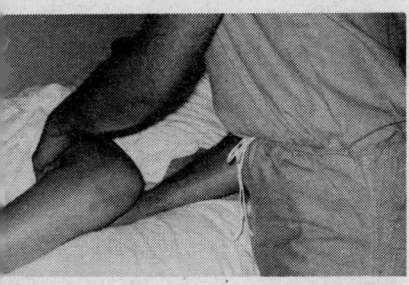

Fig. 51. Husband checking relaxation of right leg.

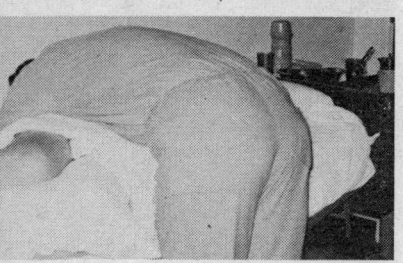

Fig. 52. A long reach for a massage of backache!

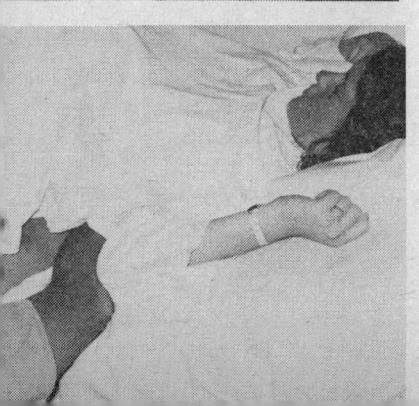

Fig. 53. "Reclining chair" position, husband still massaging backache.

lower back, and relax the pelvic area so completely that the outlet seems to be falling open of its own accord. Her husband, and an attendant as well, should test her right knee and hip joint for looseness and flexibility throughout this area.

Breathing

During labor the control of breathing plays a large part in avoiding discomfort and assisting the uterus to carry out its work. As the contractions of the first stage increase in intensity, breath is taken *more deeply* into the diaphragm but still quietly and smoothly, lips parted. *Twenty-four to twenty-eight deep breaths* may be taken in a minute (one in-and-out breath every two or three seconds, *but not more*).* The reason for this is that the uterus, which is a large, muscular organ, not only uses a great deal of oxygen to maintain its activity, but has to get rid of the carbon dioxide, the waste product of energy. Since we take in oxygen and throw off carbon dioxide through our lungs, an increased intake and output of air is an obvious corollary to uterine action.

A husband can give valuable assistance in coaching the breathing, reminding his wife to breathe deeply enough to expand the lower diaphragm and abdomen during a contraction, letting it rise and fall gently with each breath until the contraction ceases. This can be as effectively done in the lateral position as in any other. He must make sure that her breathing does not become irregular, rapid, or shallow. Such unnatural breathing patterns are signs of tension and anxiety that deprive the uterus of needed oxygen and cause discomfort. A watch with a second hand will help him keep her breathing under control. After each contraction, he should remind her to take one or two full, deep breaths, to cleanse the lungs of "used" air.

The points to remember for comfortable contractions are to

---

* Faster breathing techniques may lead to hyperventilation.

keep the abdomen, pelvic area, hip and thigh muscles and joints completely slack, while lying in the left lateral position. As the uterus comes into action, deep in-and-out breaths are to be taken, causing the abdomen to rise and fall gently. And while the woman should keep her eyes open so she can follow instructions, her face must remain relaxed, her lips parted, her jaw slack. There must be no frown or puckered brow, no screwed-up eyes, no pursed lips. There is no need for these exhibitions, for they do more harm than good and cause tension elsewhere, with consequent discomfort.

Relaxation

Relaxation during the first-stage contractions has the most astonishing effect. If the patient has been sympathetically treated and well instructed, she should have no difficulty whatever in avoiding all pain during the first stage of normal labor. It may be that it will not be easy for her, during the last part of the first stage, to avoid discomfort, but the calmer she is the more relaxed she will become. It is difficult to relax when under the influence of strong emotional disturbance.

When a physician has acquired for his patient some degree of relaxation, he should remember not to be too ambitious and expect too much of her. But occasionally he will have the absolute delight of finding a woman who becomes adept at relaxing. When he does, if everything else is normal, he should call in his medical friends, gather the students around, collect the nurses, and let them come and see a real natural labor. I have had many such cases. Some of them have appeared to be lying as if in a daydream from the beginning of their labor until the end. Their relaxation was so complete that they became almost oblivious to the fact of parturition, and, at the end of the first stage, relaxation during the contractions of the so-called pain period of labor enabled them to pass through it without discomfort. They then automatically brought into play the muscles of expulsion as the second stage began, but continued to lie in a completely relaxed state when not pushing.

The idea of pain-relievers and pain to such completely relaxed women is quite absurd. It does not enter their minds. They have no desire for it, for they do not have pain. But they understand what is said to them, listen, and carry out instructions in full cooperation.

Discomfort

No woman should be allowed to suffer greater discomfort in labor than she is willing to endure for her child's sake. In my experience the use of anesthesia presents no difficulty. If there are clinical indications, the signs and symptoms determine the most suitable method of pain relief. But even with the array of simple and effective methods of pain relief available, considerable experience is required in order to obtain the desired results. It should not be overlooked that if any reagents are used contrary to clinical indication, or at the wrong time in labor, serious trouble may ensue. The most important factor, therefore, in the use of analgesia and anesthesia in childbirth is the skill, experience, and judgment of the attending physician. Without these nothing is either safe *or effective*.* No reagent of any kind, of course, should be given without the doctor's written order, specific for that particular patient.

TRANSITION

Just before the cervix is fully dilated, that is to say, stretched wide enough to allow the baby to pass through into the vaginal portion of the birth canal, certain changes occur. In about 50 percent of women the ultimate stretching of this

* Bowes, *et al.*, *The Effects of Obstetrical Medication on Fetus and Infant*. Monograph of the Society for Research in Child Development (Chicago: University of Chicago Press, 35, no. 4, 1970).

rim of muscle tissue at the outlet of the uterus gives rise to a backache over the sacrum or bottom end of the spine. The pain is caused by the stretching of the tissues but is referred to the lower back and felt as backache. This ache can be relieved by firm pressure of the hand of husband or attendant, or by slow, heavy rubbing over the lower back and sacrum.

The contractions are strong at this point, for it takes powerful contractions on the part of the uterus to pull the circular muscles completely back over the baby's head. Yet this is a most important time for the mother to be able to relax with each contraction and not oppose it.

The temporary discomfort of the backache often is accompanied by a second change in the attitude of the woman toward her labor. Not infrequently it is the first time she has been aware of any physical uneasiness, and it awakens in her mind many fears lest this backache resolve into a more severe pain. Fear definitely assaults the minds of many women just before full dilatation of the cervix.

This backache, however, only persists for about nine to twelve contractions. A woman should be informed of that, for a temporary discomfort is much more easily borne than one which is likely to persist. She should also be told to concentrate upon the depth and rapidity of her breathing, breathing through her mouth, her face relaxed. It is possible to relax efficiently in spite of the fact that breathing is quicker and drawn deeper into the diaphragm.

Now for the first time vague signs of pressure, those early symptoms of the second stage, appear. Even a well-prepared woman can be confused. She needs guidance, coaching, encouragement. She needs the skill of her helpers in controlling her deep, even, breathing as she relaxes with each contraction. At this point, it is more comfortable for the patient to turn onto her back and be propped up in the reclining chair position, her back raised, and knees raised and resting on supports. Her head and shoulders should rest on a pillow, her neck relaxed and head turned slightly to the side and tilted back a bit, her arms and legs remaining completely limp during contractions.

As this transition from the first to the second stage of labor develops, there may come an irresistible desire to bear down and push the baby from the uterus. If the desire to push comes during a contraction, the patient should remain relaxed and pant softly or blow out through her mouth to keep from pushing, until the desire passes. *She should never bear down until she is unable to avoid it.*

Summary of First-Stage Labor*

I. *Onset of Labor*
   1. Rhythmic contractions. Leaking of waters. The "show."
   2. Expectancy, exhilaration, and animation.
   3. Doctor is called. Any normal, desired activity is continued, relaxing just during contractions. Go to hospital when doctor directs.

II. *Early First-Stage Labor*
   1. Cervix dilates to 3/5ths.
   2. Cheerfulness, followed by temporary anxiety. Desire for companionship. Labor taken more seriously.
   3. Relaxation in any comfortable position during contractions, "sleep" breathing, ample liquid intake, rest or sleep as desired.

III. *Late First-Stage Labor*
   1. Cervix dilates to 4/5ths, contractions stronger, more frequent.
   2. Temporary anxiety again, caused by strengthening contractions. Can be overcome by reassurance and careful coaching.
   3. Complete relaxation in left lateral position during contractions, allowing "sleep" breathing to change to slightly deeper "work" breathing, evenly and quietly, not more than 24 to 28 breaths a minute. Complete relaxation between contractions.

IV. *Transition*
   1. Cervix dilates to completion.
   2. Acute sensitiveness to words and noises, bright lights, or other disturbances. Backache in over half the women, causing some anxiety. Relaxation gradually becoming difficult, with the change in breathing required for expulsive contractions causing some confusion.
   3. Some relief of backache, achieved by firm rubbing of the sacrum. "Work" breathing kept at an even, moderate pace.

* Key: (1) Physical symptoms; (2) emotional symptoms; (3) position and aids to comfort

Change made from the left lateral to "reclining chair" position, sitting with the back at a 45° angle, knees supported. Any desire to push resisted by breathing short, rapid breaths in and out until the momentary urge passes. Relaxation maintained between and *during* contractions.

7

Birth: Second-Stage Labor

Once the second stage begins a woman not only gives the appearance of, but often expresses, great relief. She is now able to help. Her backache disappears, things are making progress, and soon, in an hour or two, as she should be told, her baby will be born if she works with a will.

EARLY SECOND-STAGE LABOR

When the second stage is established the routine of labor changes. The patient should not be allowed to push violently at first, but merely to hold her breath and exert a little pressure with each contraction, leaning forward and pressing down on the top of the uterus (fig. 54). It is a great mistake to wear a woman out with violent muscular effort in the beginning of the second stage of labor. The uterus will do its work perfectly well with a minimum of assistance.

Pushing with second-stage contractions requires physical effort; therefore it is obvious that relaxation during contractions must be discontinued. But as soon as a contraction has ended the mother should lean back comfortably against a raised back support, close her eyes, take one or two deep in-and-out breaths, and completely relax *between* contractions (fig. 55). These contractions may come every five or six minutes at first, but gradually at shorter intervals.

After ten or twelve contractions it will be observed that the woman becomes very drowsy between them. This state of inattention to surroundings is nature's way of preventing pain by keeping the mother relaxed. It is not, however, for the purpose of taking pain away, because very few women have any physical discomfort at this phase of the second stage. It is the means by which a woman's mind and body are completely rested, creating a condition in which the body can *recuperate with great rapidity between its violent efforts*. She is thereby prepared for each succeeding contraction without becoming exhausted. It is essential therefore that *absolute quiet* be maintained in the labor ward.* Inconsequent conversation between attendants, clumsy movements, heavy footsteps, and banging doors are unforgivable sins in the presence of a woman advanced in labor.

Subdued lighting is important as an aid to her relaxation. Many women sleep between contractions, while others remain quietly unresponsive to their surroundings. Sometimes it is difficult to make them understand what is said without speaking loudly into their ears. Since they will often respond more automatically to a command given by the husband, the doctor gives the instructions and the husband relays them to his wife.

The Husband

An obstetrician should not allow the isolation of a husband to be established by his alienation from the birth of his child. His concern and his place in this family matter should be sympathetically recognized, and every effort made to bring him into close contact with the event. There is little advantage

---

* Dr. Dick-Read makes no mention of the removal of a woman to a separate room for the actual birth. This is an American custom. In most of the world it is an accepted practice to permit a mother to labor, deliver, and recover in the same bed without being moved from her room.—Ed.

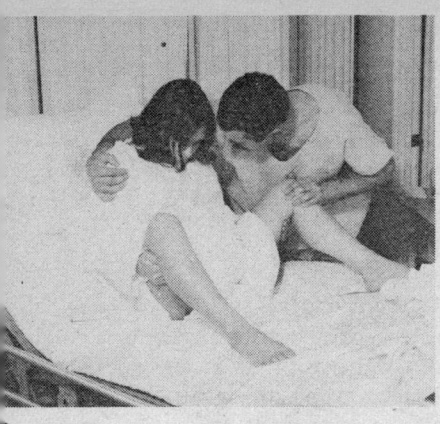

Fig. 54. Bearing down in labor room, early second stage, knees drawn up and widely apart, back rounded head bent forward.

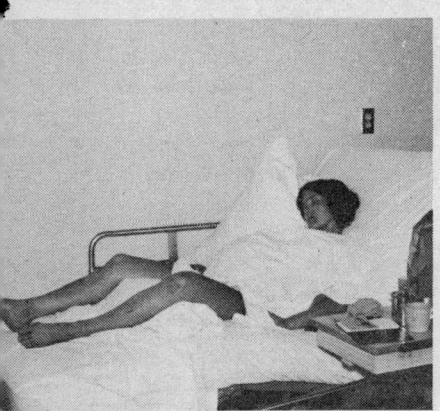

Fig. 55. Complete muscular relaxation in "reclining chair" position, between bearing-down efforts.

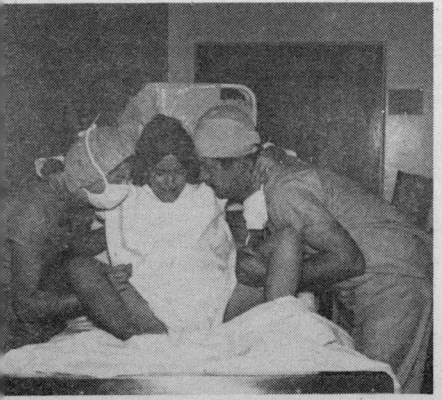

Fig. 56. Bearing down correctly, with husband and nurse assisting.

to be gained by making childbirth an incomparable delight to the woman if in so doing the husband is estranged and seeds of discord are sown in the home. Much trouble and sadness occurs from the isolation of the husband.*

Position

As soon as the second stage is under way and the mother is helping to push her baby through the birth canal, she should be placed in a semisitting position with her knees wide apart. Adopting this modified squatting posture gives the greatest freedom of muscular action to her, and also allows for the maximum size of the pelvic outlet to be obtained.

In order to achieve this position she should be propped up on a backrest to an angle of about 45 degrees. During a contraction she is to lean forward over the abdomen, with her knees drawn up beside her body, near her armpits. As she grips under her knees with her hands and pulls them outward and upward, her feet are to be supported either on the stirrups or by her attendants (fig. 56).

Other positions are adopted by the women of races whose lives habituate them to different customs. For instance, some of the Far Eastern peoples squat on their feet when their babies are delivered. Certain nomadic races kneel, giving birth to their babies very easily in that position. In some countries the horseshoe-shaped labor chair was in use until the beginning of the nineteenth century, and may well appear in modernized form; a good deal can be said in its favor.

---

* The husband will of course observe the customary aseptic techniques before accompanying his wife to the delivery room (figs. 57, 58). He will scrub, and wear appropriate operating room attire, including cap, mask and conductive shoes. He can help his wife become comfortable in the correct position on the delivery table, adjusting the backrest to her particular needs, and can help support her when she leans forward to push. He can repeat the doctors' instructions to her, remind her to take cleansing breaths after pushing, and thus become a valuable member of the birth team. In the drowsy state of second stage, a woman responds best to his familiar voice.

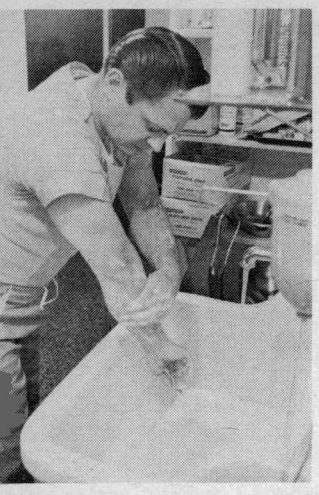

Fig. 57. Husband scrubbing before accompanying wife into birth room.

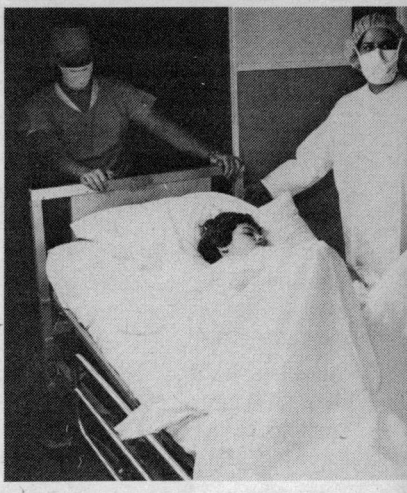

Fig. 58. Moving from labor room to birth room.

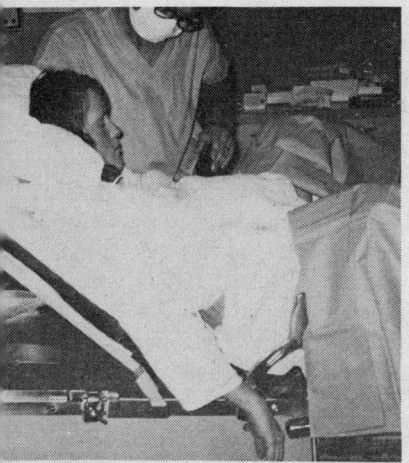

Fig. 59. Mother of twins totally relaxed between second-stage contractions.

WELL-ESTABLISHED SECOND-STAGE LABOR

Breathing

Once the pushing reflex is well established during the second stage of labor, respiration ceases while the woman leans over and bears down in an expulsive effort. At the same time the uterus is contracting firmly and the high quantity of carbon dioxide accumulating in the blood is shown by a change in the color of the woman's face as the contraction persists. She may become swarthy and cyanosed, which is a blue tint under the skin, for blood containing an excess of carbon dioxide is a dark blue-red color. Therefore, she must be trained during pregnancy to hold her breath, for by so doing she can learn to retain in her blood the slight increase of carbon dioxide without distress, and at the same time overcome the desire to let her breath go when it is advantageous to hold it.

That is why *after each expulsive contraction she is told to lean back against the backrest and take two or three controlled, full, in-and-out breaths,* thus replacing the oxygen used and clearing the lungs of carbon dioxide. Then she should completely relax and wait restfully for the next contraction in a state of peace (fig. 59).

Respiration between contractions is quiet breathing, that is, "sleep" breathing, the abdomen rising and falling slightly as the patient rests. The absence of muscle tension between contractions minimizes the need for oxygen and the formation of the waste products of tension. It also permits complete dilation of both the arteries and veins in the abdomen and pelvis, and enables a free intake of all the fuel necessary for the low state of metabolism between contractions.

Relaxation

One could not require, nor would it be possible to obtain, physical relaxation during expulsive contractions of the sec-

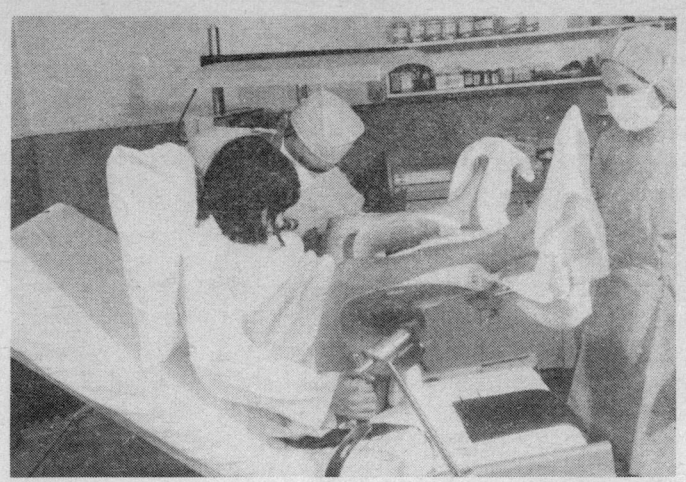

Fig. 60. Bearing down with second-stage contraction, back curved, head forward, knees wide and back toward shoulders, husband supporting shoulders.

Fig. 61. Complete relaxation against backrest between second-stage contractions, husband giving instructions.

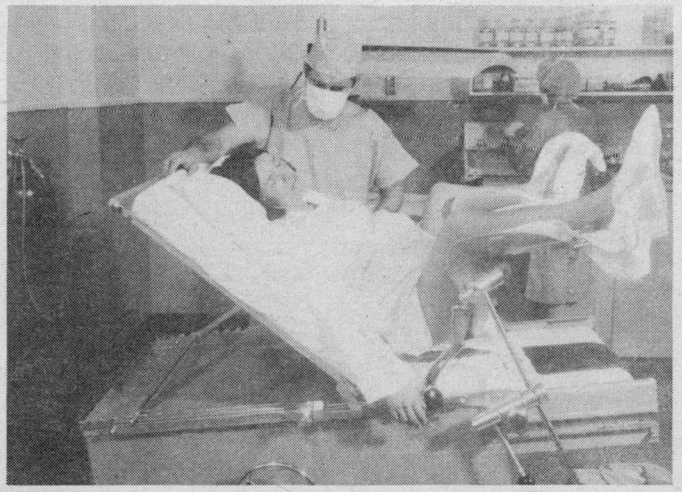

ond stage (fig. 60). The idea of nature here is that, the door being widely opened and the birth canal ready for the baby to pass through, the mother can assist the muscles of the uterus by pushing down vigorously. This requires real physical exertion, and since after each second-stage contraction the woman will be plainly out of breath, deep in-and-out breaths must be taken to quickly replace the oxygen used. Then, *between* the contractions complete relaxation is necessary, for relaxation is the most effective manner of quickly reconstituting muscle power (fig. 61).

It is usual for the membranes, the bag of waters in which the baby is contained, to have ruptured before this time. *A woman should always be reminded of the imminence of this event,* because many are alarmed by the sudden and unexpected flow of a large amount of water.

Anesthesia

There is very little, if any, discomfort in the average, properly conducted second stage of labor. During the first stage many women become bored, and a little tired of the feeling that nothing can be done. Thus a tremendous sense of relief very often fills a woman's mind as she realizes that not only can she help, but the greater effort she applies, within reason, the greater sense of comfort she will get. There is no pain with a good honest second-stage expulsive effort until the first awareness of dilatation of the perineum is felt. I am not, of course, speaking of abnormal cases, such as those in which large masses of piles come down as the head stretches the anterior wall of the rectum, but of the normal, unimpeded case in which no pathological condition is present at all.

No woman should be allowed to suffer pain in labor, and every method discovered by science should be used to prevent it. If there is true pain, anesthetics and analgesics should be exhibited at once, but the absence of severe discomfort contraindicates its use. *It is as great a crime to leave a woman alone in her agony and deny her relief from her suffering as it is to insist upon dulling the consciousness of a natural mother who desires above all things to be aware of the final reward of her efforts. Each of these two unforgivable errors is constantly committed.*

There should always be an anesthetic or analgesic apparatus at hand during labor, and if necessary the patient should be instructed in its use. Women adequately trained for natural childbirth very rarely desire anesthesia and frequently refuse its use. Women who have not had the advantage of preparing themselves to give birth may have considerable pain, which they are causing themselves; therefore analgesia and anesthesia should be used. It must be recognized, however, that 95 percent of these deprived women could have had natural labors if they had been properly prepared.

When there is a *definite abnormality,* such as disproportion or a malpresentation or one of those rare complications which must be diagnosed and treated by an experienced obstetrician, drugs and anesthetics should be adequately applied under his instructions as quickly as possible. *That is one of the greatest benefits anesthesia has brought to humanity, and when a woman suffers the pain of abnormality in childbirth it should never be withheld.*

The administration of anesthetics and analgesics should have definite indication in obstetrics as it has in every other branch of medicine or surgery. Pain is the most frequent justification; it does not matter whether the pain is secondary to fear or whether it is primarily physical. Natural childbirth mothers have no fear and therefore little discomfort. Because the discomfort is minimal few, if any, of these prepared women demand relief.

When the head gets down onto the muscles that form the floor of the pelvis, a woman often finds it difficult to relax the outlet, because she gets a sense of the passageway opening up, a new sensation to every first-time mother. If she is alarmed by this sensation and endeavors to resist as the head arrives within an inch of the outlet, contracting her pelvic floor and squeezing the vulva and rectum tightly, she runs a very good chance of having not only acute pain but also, by increasing resistant tension, a torn perineum.

At this time a definite wave of fear comes over most women, caused by this feeling of opening up below, and an uncontrollable desire to *escape*. It is important not to yield too quickly to the assumption that the woman is in pain, for this threat to her self-control is not difficult to overcome. She must be strongly reassured that she will not "burst," that the opening will not hurt as it stretches further; she must be told how to overcome the discomfort. At the next contraction she is to *concentrate and push as firmly as she can*. As soon as she exerts this *maximum* pressure, the pelvic floor becomes distended and the head rapidly passes down to the vulva without further discomfort.

CROWNING

When the head is visible and no longer slips back between contractions, what is called *crowning* has occurred. As the vulva dilates to about two inches in diameter the outlet can be felt stretching, a sensation that has been described as one of burning or bursting.

It is important that a woman *relax completely* at this time, letting her jaw fall slack and *breathing with her mouth open*. The muscles of the perineum relax as her face and mouth relax. She should be told that the sensation of bursting is a myth. The head will not tear the perineum if she is *completely relaxed,* all her muscles slack and her facial muscles relaxed, and if she breathes softly in and out through her *open mouth*. It is astonishing how large a baby will then pass through what appears to be a small vulva without any tear to the perineum at all. If, between the final second-stage contractions, after the head is adequately crowned, the attendant can persuade a woman to remain relaxed in this way, the complete absence of difficulty with which the head can be produced is surprising. I am sure that a large number of torn perineums are due to the effort of the woman to resist the oncoming head by violently contracting the muscles at the outlet. If her husband sees her close her mouth, or set it in a grim line, he should immediately remind her to relax her face and breathe through her open mouth.

As soon as the head has crowned, *all efforts to bear down should be stopped*. During contractions the uterus itself will slowly urge the child forward while the woman fully relaxes, opens her mouth, and breathes in and out quickly, to keep from pushing. In this way the vulva is gradually distended without discomfort. It must be distended gradually without any violence, for tears of the skin and even of the muscles are frequently produced unnecessarily because a woman is erroneously encouraged to bear down at this time.

BIRTH

As the head is born, it must be supported by the attendant and turned up over the pubis of the mother. Once the baby's head is born there is often a pause (fig. 62). It may cry before the shoulders arrive. With the next contraction, which again must be completely controlled by the attendant to keep the baby from moving too quickly, the baby's body emerges (fig. 63). He may ask the mother to refrain from pushing during contractions, or he may have the mother bear down very gently if the uterus requires a little assistance from the mother.

When a baby arrives under these conditions the woman, being conscious and not filled with anesthetic, often realizes that her baby has been born only after she hears it cry. A child passes through a relaxed vulva with almost complete absence of sensation to the mother. There is no doubt that with relaxation of the vulva there is also a temporary natural anesthesia of its sensory nerves.

The case of a young woman whom I attended is an example of this. As her second stage of labor began, I instructed her in how to bear down, and asked her gently to increase her efforts. Then I sent for the medical students to come observe. They seemed unable to believe that she had passed so smilingly and so comfortably through the first stage. After a few more honest contractions, the rectum bulged. Soon the head appeared, and she looked at me inquiringly and said, "Can I really stretch enough? It feels as if something must give way." I pointed out to her that this was the invariable sensation of a conscious woman, but that it was only a temporary sensation, for as the head was born it turned away from the point where she was feeling the pressure. She accepted my assurance confidently, and in three or four more contractions a large baby's head was born easily and painlessly into my hands. I told her that her baby's head had arrived and that it was a lovely child. She was unwilling to believe that I was not encouraging her by making her think the head had come when it had not, so I pointed out to her that she could feel the child's head against her thigh and also see it if she looked. She was incredulous as she looked down and saw her child.

I asked her to bear down gently so that the rest of the child could be born. She said, "Tell me at once if it is a boy. We are longing for a boy." And so I was able to lift up to her a crying, beautiful baby boy of eight pounds one ounce, as we soon discovered upon weighing him. Her joy was indeed a picture to behold. There was no question of pain, she had been instructed how to use the inhalant but had refused, assuring us that there was nothing in this experience but the most unqualified delight. At first she was too excited to speak as she took the child in her hands, but then she said, "I must look carefully—it is difficult to believe I have a boy. It is wonderful!" And as she laughed and fondled her child, tears of joy rolled down her cheeks.

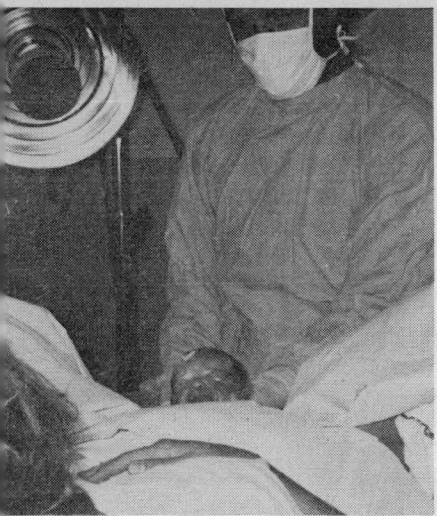

Fig. 62. Baby's head is born, supported upward by attending physician.

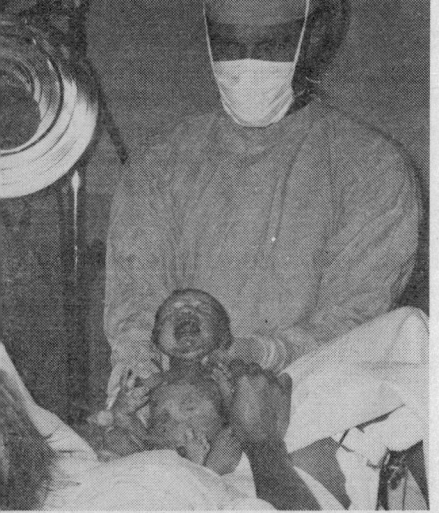

Fig. 63. Baby's body is born, supported upward, over the pubic bone and toward the mother, by attending physician.

Summary of Second-Stage Labor*

I. *Early Second-Stage Labor*
   1. Expulsive reflex not strong. Backache ceases.
   2. Temporary revival of personality and determination.
   3. Semisitting position on birth table, backrest at 45° angle. Breath holding during contractions followed by one or two deep breaths. "Sleep" breathing and relaxation between contractions. Leaning forward to push, arms out at right angles, knees drawn back toward shoulders. Leaning back to rest.

II. *Well-Established Second-Stage Labor*
   1. Head progressing down birth canal to pelvic cavity. Expulsive effort stronger. No discomfort but hard work.
   2. Woman's true self evident. Sometimes discretion and discrimination is "low." Increased drowsiness between contractions. Sudden impatience and desire to escape as head reaches pelvic floor.
   3. To overcome discomfort, take a deep breath, hold it, and *push as firmly as possible.* A partial expulsive effort may seem uncomfortable, a complete expulsive effort overcomes the discomfort.

III. *Birth*
   1. Stretching and thinning of the perineum. Crowning, and burning feeling around the vulva temporarily, disappearing as stretching increases.
   2. Exasperation as the burning is felt, discretion low, but response to the encouragement of attendants. As head is born, drowsiness replaced by mental alertness and incredulity. Weariness vanishes.
   3. Perineum to be kept *fully relaxed.* No bearing down as the head or shoulders emerge, but rapid in-and-out breathing to keep from pushing.

---

* Key: (1) Physical symptoms; (2) emotional symptoms; (3) position and aids to comfort

8

Immediate Newborn Period: Third-Stage Labor

In natural childbirth, once the baby is born, there is no need for relaxation. Here we get the beautiful *tension* of satisfaction. The sympathetic nervous system sweeps in with all its joys and its pleasing emotions, and so there is no desire for relaxation. The strain and weariness of muscular effort are swept from the mother's memory by the sound and sight of her newborn child, and this stimulates the uterus into the action of the third stage.

When the child is first born it is my custom to lift him up for the mother to see (figs. 64, 65), then lay him flat on the bed between his mother's thighs and wait until pulsation of the cord has ceased before severing it. Sometimes it may be four or five minutes before pulsation fades, during which time the baby is covered with warm towels.

If there has been a small nick of skin which the obstetrician considers will heal better with one or two stitches, these can be inserted while the perineum is still numb, with a minimum of discomfort to the woman and without any anesthetic. The woman is asked to relax while they are being inserted. I use a semicircular needle of an inch, or an inch and a quarter in its greatest diameter, passing the point of the needle quickly through the skin at right angles to the surface both in and out.

This must be done at once, however, because the natural

anesthesia of the vulva disappears in a very few minutes. If it is delayed for a quarter of an hour or more, then some local anesthetic, such as 1 percent novocaine, should be injected into the area through which the ligature is passed. These stitches are not tied until the placenta has arrived, and it is interesting to note that the tying, if not very gently done, is likely to prove much more uncomfortable than the insertion. This relative natural anesthesia of the perineum persisting in the early part of the third stage of labor is worthy of note, for it permits immediate suture, if needed. It is probably true also that lacerated surfaces brought into apposition before coagulation has occurred heal more quickly and more firmly than those which remain open before they are repaired. If an episiotomy is performed and a more extensive repair is required, the routine procedure of the attendant obstetrician will be adopted.

As soon as the cord is severed, the child is wrapped in warmed towels and given to his mother to hold. Some have an immediate desire to put the baby to breast. This contact stimulates, by direct reflex, strong contractions and retractions of the uterus, thus hastening separation of the placenta and the closing of the blood vessels in the part of the uterus to which it was attached.

This may be confirmed if one's hand is placed lightly on the abdomen as the baby is put to the mother's breast. Thus one of the most important benefits of the physical contact of the newborn with its mother is this rapid separation of the afterbirth, and the absence of any excessive hemorrhage. Those of us who are aware of the results of the mismanagement of the third stage of labor can adequately assess the importance of this phenomenon.

After the mother has held her baby for a few minutes, he is placed in a warm crib beside her. She is given a hot or cold drink with plenty of sugar, to replenish her energy and the loss of fluid in her system. Many women have violent *shivering attacks,* at about this time, which are alarming if not ex-

THIRD-STAGE LABOR 81

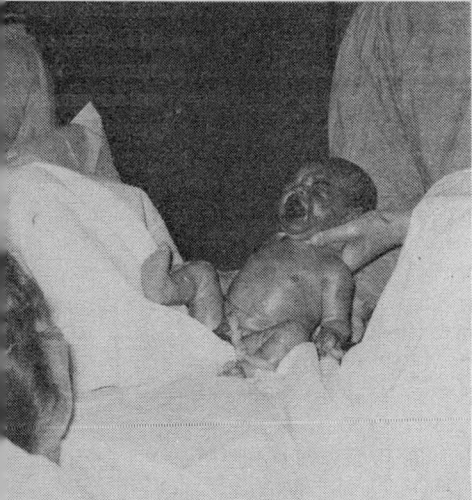

Fig. 64. Attending physician holds baby up for mother to see.

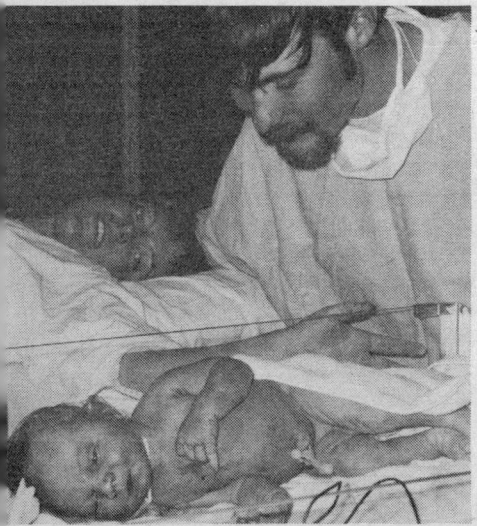

Fig. 65. Proud parents admiring newborn.

plained. Shivering is the natural method of replacing some of the body heat lost when the waters, the baby, and finally the placenta leave the mother's body, and is equivalent to shivering when we feel cold, the producing of maximum warmth with minimum exertion. The mother should be helped to become comfortably warm again. (Shivering experienced earlier in labor is a nervous reaction to emotional states, causing cold sensations and excessive muscular tension. It rarely occurs in a trained, relaxed woman, unless the room is too cold or her covers insufficient for warmth.)

It should not be overlooked that many women believe the delivery of the afterbirth to be an event of considerable severity and discomfort. Therefore the care of a woman's mind during this twenty minutes or so continues to be important.

She need not relax, but may be asked to bear down gently with these painless, miniature second-stage type contractions. Not infrequently a mother will expel the afterbirth without any assistance from the physician, and with a minimum of blood loss. This is possible because of the absence of either exhaustion or shock in a natural birth.

The placenta is a spongy, soft organ that varies in size with the size and weight of the child. Usually oval or circular in shape, it measures from six inches to nine inches wide and about three-fourths of an inch deep at the center, thinning off at the edges. The average weight is about one pound. It shapes itself very easily to the contour of the birth canal and is passed without difficulty.

Years ago it was unheard of that a woman should wish to see the afterbirth. Today nearly every mother who watches her baby born asks me to show her the placenta. (A few women have no desire to look at it.) This I do if she requests it (figs. 66, 67), pointing out the bag in which the infant, now lying peacefully in her arms or by her side, developed and became a perfect little human being (fig. 68). I show her the cord and its attachments, and the manner in which substances are

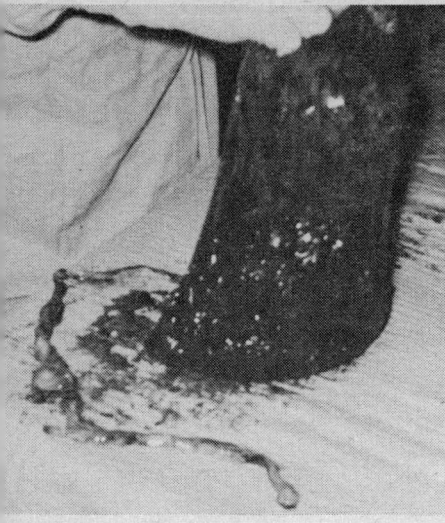

Fig. 66. Physician showing parents the placenta in the membranes.

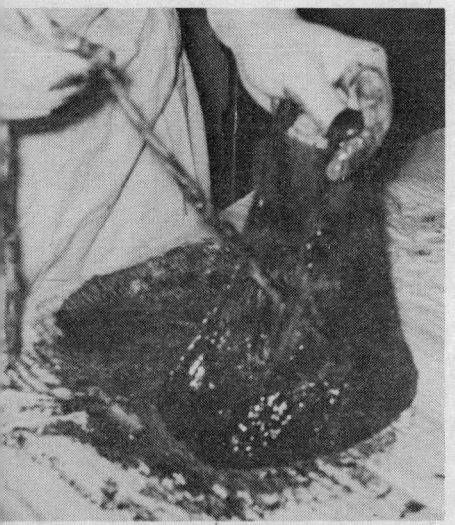

Fig. 67. Physician showing parents the membranes in which the baby lay, and the cord attached to the placenta.

filtered from the maternal blood to build the body, mind, and nature of her child. The amazing powers of selecting and rejecting substances that the placenta has for the fetus at its different stages of growth is remarkable. Its capacity for selecting the correct food in balanced quantities and refusing to admit much, though not all, that might be harmful, makes the intelligent mind appreciate the incalculable genius of creation in all its phases and designs.

"Madam," I tell my patient, "when man can make one of these, he will have reached the footstool of the Creator. As I hold this discarded mass in my hand, I am humbled by the limitations of science." Such references create respect and help us visualize childbirth in its correct perspective. By speaking of the placenta in these terms, the importance of judicious diet and the influence of harmful chemicals that may pass into the baby's blood can be more fully appreciated.

After the placenta is expelled, the nurse then swabs the vulva and perineum carefully with an anesthetic and a sterile napkin is adjusted to receive what is known as the *lochia*. So labor ends, and the woman, accompanied by her husband, is returned to her bed (fig. 69), where she is given a cup of tea, orange juice, or other nourishment and made comfortable to rest from her exertions. The newborn baby should remain with his mother.

THIRD-STAGE LABOR

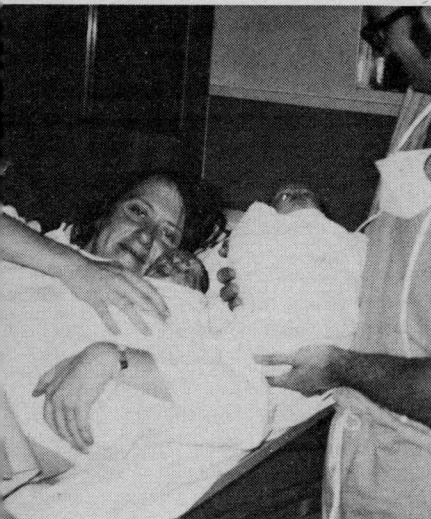

Fig. 68. Twins!

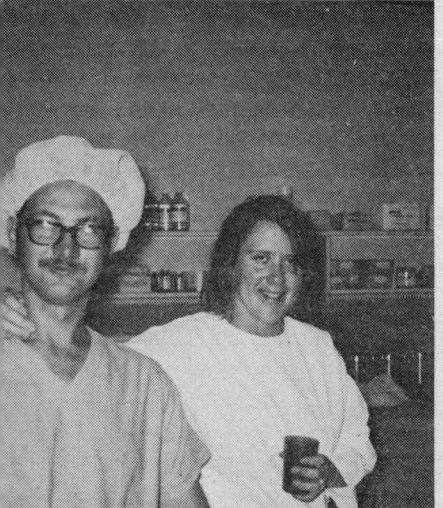

Fig. 69. Walking to room with husband after giving birth to twins, orange juice in hand.

Editors' Addendum

INSTRUCTIONS ON THE IMMEDIATE ROUTINE CARE OF THE NEWBORN*

1. The baby is kept horizontal at about the level of the placenta until cord pulsations have ceased.
   a. During this time, first nasal then pharyngeal aspiration is accomplished.
   b. The nurse will remind the attending physician at both sixty seconds and five minutes for Apgar ratings.
   c. It is to be noted that the baby's head is not to be lower than the feet (to prevent excess intracranial pressure), nor is the baby to be held for any significant length of time above or below the level of the placenta until after the cessation of cord pulsation.
   d. The notable exceptions to the above rules would be in the premature infant or in the Rh or ABO sensitization, when early clamping of the cord is indicated.
   e. In all mothers who are Rh-negative, and/or previously sensitized, a cord blood specimen, including Coombs, Rh, and type is to be taken. If the mother is known to be already sensitized, further specimens of oxalated and whole blood obtained for other study is indicated, such as bilirubin and hemoglobin determination. If a mother who is Rh-negative has an Rh-positive baby, the mother then becomes a candidate for Rho Gam injection.

2. As soon as the cord has stopped pulsating and has been clamped and severed, the baby is immediately transferred to a prewarmed IMI warmer or similar type birth room warmer, and skin thermostat applied.

3. Identification of infant is performed in the birth room and checked by both the nurse and the physician.

4. 1% silver nitrate is placed in each eye.

* See also *Standards and Recommendations for Hospital Care of Newborn Infants* (American Academy of Pediatrics, 1966).

THIRD-STAGE LABOR

5. Vitamin K is given I.M. to each newborn baby, in the birth room when possible.

6. If the mother has been prepared to start early nursing, she may do so on the delivery table by moving the hood of the IMI warmer over herself and keeping the skin thermostat attached to the baby, to control and register the temperature of the baby and maintain newborn body warmth. With the exception of a problem in the newborn, the newborn is to be placed as close to the mother as possible for as long as possible before being transferred to the nursery.

7. The baby is not to be removed from the birth room until his condition is considered normal or the attending physician so orders.

8. The only cleansing of the baby is to be the cleaning off of blood and/or meconium with lukewarm water. At times, it may take a small amount of baby oil to clean adherent areas of meconium. All vernix caseosa is to remain on the baby. In order to keep the baby close to the mother as long as possible, it is preferred that the baby not be returned to the nursery until the mother has been returned to her postpartum bed, at which time the baby should be returned to the mother for rooming-in. The exceptions to this are when the mother is recovering from an anesthetic, or she does not wish the baby, or the doctor requests that the baby not be taken back to the mother at that time.

9. All mothers on a childbirth training program and listed as early nursing mothers should have their baby brought to them as soon as possible after the mother has returned to her postpartum bed, and remain with the mother as much as possible during the first twenty-four hours of life.

10. Whenever possible during this first twenty-four hours the husband should be permitted to be with his wife and to hold their baby. He should first have pHisoHex or equivalent scrub of his hands and wear gown and mask during this period. No other visitors are permitted when the baby is with his mother.

9

Natural Childbirth in Emergency

There are times when we all have to face unexpected emergency, and it is our reaction to it that is often more important than the sudden unexpected occurrence or situation with which we are confronted.

Women all over the world are, and may continue to be, caught in the emergency of unexpected labor—if only because they are alone at home or in the country or, as I have seen several times, in a public place or vehicle. Labor is not a frightening incident in the life of a woman if she has learned what goes on and how her body produces the child when it is ready to leave its mother's womb.

What can a woman do when and if in circumstances of unexpected emergency her labor begins, with no competent person to help her, and perhaps only herself to help her child safely into the world? If she has no knowledge of her own natural processes and how to assist and not hinder their performance, she creates many difficulties and much discomfort to herself, and perhaps also for her child. A known and well-proven scientific fact is that nothing disturbs the course of natural labor more than fear. Fear is caused and intensified by ignorance. The first need, then, is for the woman in such circumstances to be prepared in advance by knowledge and understanding of how to give birth to her child.

When the baby is ready to be born it lies comfortably in the uterus or womb with its *head downward,* for it is usual and best for babies to dive, not step, into the world. The baby announces its coming arrival in three ways—by a *show* of mucus or blood from the outlet of the birth canal, by a *leaking* of water from the uterus, or by *rhythmical contractions,* which increase in frequency and in strength.

The first two of these warnings, in the absence of the strong contractions of the uterus, usually give plenty of time to prepare for the baby's arrival. But under the stress of accident or the threat of death-dealing danger, as in time of war, the intense defensive reaction to paralyzing fear is almost complete relaxation and inactivity of the muscles that control the passage of the baby from the womb. Under these circumstances labor is often what we term "precipitate," and the baby arrives with very little discomfort or difficulty to the mother. Terror-caused paralysis of the muscles of the pelvic floor, allowing spontaneous evacuation of the bowel and urinary bladder, is well known, and at the end of pregnancy the same reaction to terror may occur with the uterus. This unusual state is the reverse of the fear-tension-pain syndrome.

When the intensity of fear diminishes and brings conscious realization of being in labor, women resist the effort of expulsion and thereby create a state of tension by opposing the muscles that are contracting to push the baby out. This is the reaction of emotional stress. *There is a very real difference between the emergency of precipitate labor due to external stress,* with the primitive defense reaction to violent and imminent destruction, *and the labor of a woman in fear of labor itself.* The defensive reaction in cases of external fright is one of emotional and physical paralysis, but in the fear of labor alone it is one of emotional and physical resistance to the work of the uterus. I have seen in trenches, on shell-swept plains, and in the rubble of bombed cities women in such emotional terror that they have lost all voluntary control, and have compared them with women in perfectly safe surroundings, frightened by the process of labor itself. These women suffer even though under the care of well-meaning attendants, whose tender ministrations and sympathetic manner reveal that they expect their patient to be in pain, and thus add to her tension and discomfort.

The most important thing to remember, then, is that it is *fear* of pain that produces all the severe and unbearable suffering of labor. In an emergency, a *calm* woman who remains in control of her actions will have little discomfort as she awaits the progression of the natural events about which she has learned.

During labor a woman should pass urine from time to time, in order to keep her urinary bladder empty. This should be done in a squatting position at any reasonable place, according to the dilemma in which she may find herself.

Then, wherever she is, in a wayside ditch or a ruin-covered cellar, in a stranger's house, a caravan, or tent, she should find a place to *sit down and lean her back against*—wall, bank, or any available support. She should pull up her knees and rest her buttocks on a folded coat, a bunch of leaves, or anything that will lift her slightly off the ground. She should *not lie down on her side or her back, but sit* as near as possible in a squatting position, taking the weight of her body upon her buttocks. If left alone in labor, she may escape one of the greatest causes of trouble, which is interference by those around who, being kind but misinformed, feel they must *do* something for her. The safest medical attendant in such an emergency is nature, by whom woman has been marvelously equipped for this purpose. The baby is not to be interfered with by its mother's mind or a volunteer assistant's hand. Just courage and patience are required, and faith in God, if she is a believer, to produce a healthy baby and be a happy mother.

As the woman sits and waits patiently for the baby, she will soon feel a desire to push down. At first the effort to push must be very gentle. She should only take a deep breath and hold it, without pushing. There may be some backache, but it will soon pass. If there is no one there to rub her back she must relax and try to put it out of her mind, for the backache will soon disappear. When the desire to bear down becomes too strong to resist, she may begin to push firmly, but not too hard, and without expecting immediate results. If it is her first baby, it may take one and a half to two hours of expulsive effort before the baby appears. Sometimes two or three deep breaths, in and out, may be taken during one contraction, if it is too long for one breath alone. Breathe in, hold and push, breathe out and in, hold and push.

As the contraction fades she will relax sleepily, first taking two deep in and out breaths, then quietly resting until the next effort begins. Her drowsiness may be so deep that her mind is concentrated only on the one task of producing her child. I have seen women during air raids who, although by nature nervous people, were not disturbed by the noise or the flashes of bombs that rocked the walls about us. On one occasion, being disconcerted myself by the volume and proximity of missiles, I was slow to notice the onset of my twenty-two-year-old patient's next contraction. She said testily, "Another push, doctor. Come on, don't worry about the noise!"

Just before the head can be seen some women have a strong desire to "escape" the impending birth. When this occurs the woman should remember to ignore the feeling and *push firmly* for the next two or at the most three contractions. Such concentrated expulsive efforts to help the contraction will quickly overcome the temporary discomfort and desire to escape. Shortly after that the hair on the baby's head will show at the outlet. If there is a looking glass handy, so the mother can see her baby, it will help her take an active interest in helping him arrive. She will then concentrate upon the baby and his arrival and forget thoughts of her own well-being. The second or expulsive stage of labor need not be painful if the mother is in the correct squatting position, keeping her outlet relaxed and pushing properly with the contractions, though it may be hard work for the birth of a first baby. This stage is to be a conscious, controlled, and painless repetition of pushing to urge the baby forward as he moves through the natural twists and turns, flexions and extensions of the head that prevent damage to both mother and baby.

As the head starts to distend the vulva, a feeling of burning of the labia or lips of the outlet may alarm her. She must realize that it will quickly disappear *if* she does not squeeze up against it. The outlet must be relaxed and allowed to bulge as it will. But she *must not bear down* any more. Instead, she should breathe short breaths in and out, letting the abdominal muscles stay relaxed, allowing the uterus itself to urge the child slowly forward in a relatively painless birth of the head.

At this time she will have lost her drowsiness, and will be able to adjust her position, leaning back at an angle of 45 degrees—about halfway between flat and upright. With contractions she should pull her knees up and, with her hands, hold them wide open and at right angles to her body, with her feet resting on whatever support is handy.

As the baby emerges into the world face downward, the woman should lean over and put one hand on the area between the anus and the vaginal opening, so that the forehead and face of the child pass gently into her waiting hand. She can thus support her baby's head as it arrives, directing it *upward* toward her abdomen. Under no circumstances should she pull the baby out straight before her! She must remember to *help the baby upward and over the bone of the front of the pelvis,* using her second hand to support the baby's body as it emerges. Lifting the baby upward helps prevent tearing of the outlet.

If she is alone or with inexperienced people, she must not become excited or hurried. Slowness, quietness, and gentleness are the qualities of a good delivery. The crying baby is then to be laid flat on the ground, his head still supported in her hand, until the cord that joins the infant to her ceases to pulsate or throb. It will shrink and become pale and limp. By this time the placenta or afterbirth may have separated from the womb and be in the vaginal canal.

As soon as the cord has stopped pulsating and is long enough for the woman to lift the child without any pull on the cord, she should put the child to breast, raising the child gently with one hand under his head and the other under his hips. Cradling him so that he lies level along her arm she should allow him to grasp the nipple. If he will not take it as most do, she should gently rub his mouth and nose against the nipple, to stimulate her uterus.

Soon contractions will begin again, and the second stage of labor is then repeated, in a diminutive form, for the birth of the placenta, the third stage. If the afterbirth does not come of its own accord, the mother can keep the baby supported on one arm and place her hand on her abdomen above the uterus, which will be felt as a coconut-sized lump reaching just above the navel. If she presses gently on the abdomen with the palm of her hand, and then gives one or two sharp coughs, the afterbirth may come out easily.

In emergency labor the cord should not be cut until after the afterbirth comes away. Until then the baby is kept warm in its mother's clothing, either on the ground beside her or in her arms, preferably held to the breast. When the afterbirth has been expelled, it is to be wrapped up with the baby until experienced medical help is available.

Whatever clothing is available may be used for the baby and for the mother. As little as possible should be put over the birth canal outlet, which must not be touched with unwashed hands if this can be avoided, although emergency labor seldom results in infection.

Most women, after the labor is completed, are able to walk with their babies to a place where clothing and cleanliness may be obtained, and perhaps medical aid and advice.

The *dignity and control of childbirth* can be maintained even in circumstances incredibly different from our accepted standards. I have attended women in many strange places and circumstances and know that this is true. A woman must remember that faith is not only an ethical and emotional acquisition. It is also a state of mind, which creates within the body physical harmony in the activities of living that maintain the highest standard of health and resistance to disease.

10

Care of the Newborn

A newborn baby remains part of its mother just as much after birth as it was while *in utero*. Indeed, the added association of personality and behavior brings them even closer together. When a baby is born it is equipped by nature with the means of survival in relation to its mother.

In the absence of experience it does not interpret incidents in the adventure of living with adult understanding. Its physical demands are for food, warmth, and rest. Its awareness to things and people about it develops rapidly, however, and within a few hours of birth it seeks security in the widest sense. In the early days of a baby's life security implies the provision of the essentials for survival and protection from outside injurious influences. *For that security a newborn baby turns to its mother.*

BODY CONTACT

When a child is born the mother should hold it and fondle it immediately. Some mothers have the desire to put the baby to the breast. This initial skin-to-skin contact of warmth (figs. 70, 71, 72) between the mother and her child has a most salutary influence upon the progress and behavior of them both. After the mother returns to her bed, the baby is placed in a crib beside her. Knowing her child is there, she does not worry about it. She feels that her child is secure. Whenever she desires she can put the baby to her breast. For not only do breasts have the supreme function of lactation, they are also the ultimate manifestation of the mother-child relationship. As surely as the umbilical cord sustains the vital unity of the mother with her intrauterine fetus, so the nipple retains that mystic union with the child that is no longer within her. In those peaceful moments the infant floods its mother's mind in meditation, which brings reality to her most cherished dreams. His restlessness is quieted and his awareness of others stimulated through this physical and affectionate contact. An older baby often pats and fondles the breasts as he nurses, and stops to smile at his mother. Through her breast they are unified in extrauterine life as closely as in the months of gestation.

After the baby has been put to the breast it is held and cuddled, becoming familiar with the mother's ways while she herself becomes familiar with his. When a mother fondles and cuddles her baby as it nestles and nuzzles against her breast and in her arms, she is unconsciously laying a foundation of that mutual confidence and companionship from which all that is best in human nature develops.

The baby is then replaced in the crib by her bedside. Infants treated in this way are peaceful and quiet and very rarely disturb their mothers by crying.

COLOSTRUM

When a child is put to the breast shortly after birth he gets no milk, but there is a substance known as *colostrum* that exudes from a well-prepared nipple. There is still much to be learned about this valuable, thick fluid. We know that it contains substances that produce within the infant immunities to certain bacteria that might cause diseases. It contains a certain amount of milk globules and cells containing fat, which are called *colostrum corpuscles,* but the actual value of these to the baby is not yet fully known. Colostrum seems to have a beneficial effect upon the baby's bowels, helping to expel the

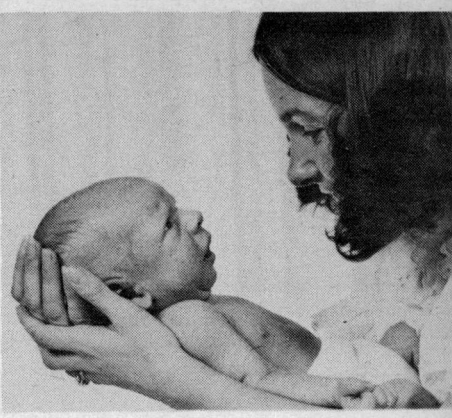

Fig. 70. Stimulation of infant through mother's hands.

meconium that is contained in the intestines of the newborn. It may be of help in breaking down the mucus in his throat when he nurses immediately after birth, by stimulating the swallowing reflex or causing him to cough before he can swallow. Colostrum may also provide enzymes for protein metabolism.

Colostrum is also of great use to the breast and nipple of the mother, for the suckling of the baby helps to stimulate the activity of the glands by which the milk is secreted. By the third day or less after the baby has been put to the breast, these milk glands become enlarged, filling the ducts leading from the breast to the nipple, of which there are about twenty. Since the baby has drawn away the thick colostrum from these ducts, the milk flow is much more quickly and easily established without engorgement, for *where the infant feeds there will be food*.

Nature provides the newborn infant with a considerable amount of fat. During the day or two before the milk is secreted in the breast, this fat in his own system is absorbed as his own natural nutrition. It is largely this provision of food within itself that accounts for his loss of weight until the mother's milk supply is established. I certainly do not advise

SKIN-TO-SKIN CONTACT

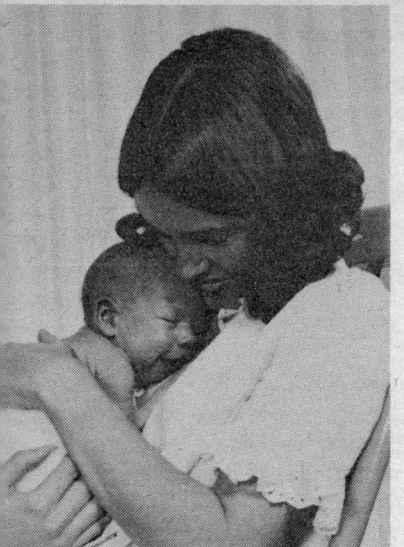

Fig. 71. Newborn maternal closeness.

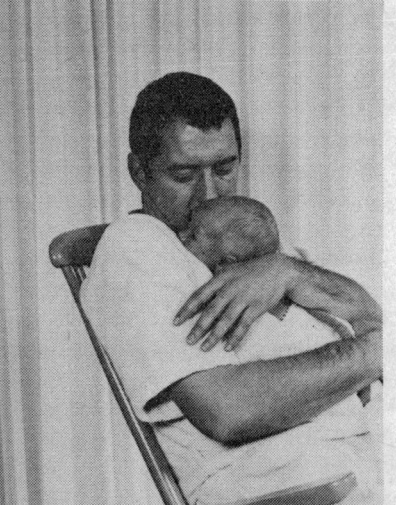

Fig. 72. Skin-to-skin with Daddy, too!

giving the baby any prescription before the natural food is available. It has enough nourishment in its own body to live comfortably until the milk supply is adequately stimulated. Not infrequently its desire to take the breast is decreased if it has supplementary or "pity" feeds, and this delays further the establishment of his mother's milk supply in an easily accessible flow.

FEEDING ON DEMAND

A child does not wish to nurse continuously. At first, when hungry, he will swallow as rapidly as possible, but he must rest. Although he does not relinquish his hold on the nipple he will stop taking milk for a short time. If he appears to be drifting into sleep, a gentle touch on the upper lip with the mother's finger will restimulate his sucking reflex.

Although it is not strictly accurate to say that the infant sucks the milk from the breast, we will use this term for the sake of simplicity. In reality, he presses the milk out by closing his mouth on the nipple with a squeezing action. The only real sucking is the action of the baby's tongue in lifting the nipple up to his palate.

An infant takes nearly all his food in the first four or five minutes, and if he becomes lazy he should be taken off the breast. This can be done without discomfort to the mother by lightly compressing the baby's nostrils so that he opens his mouth to breathe.

A newborn baby requires feeding again as soon as its last meal has been digested. One will take a large amount, and four or five hours pass before he feels he wants more and cries to gain the mother's attention to his hunger. Others may take smaller amounts, or have a more rapid digestion, and will cry after three hours or even less. The demand in a baby's voice is recognizable from all other cries, and a mother quickly learns the difference between the cry of hunger, the cry of colic, the grumble of an uncomfortable diaper, or the irregular bursts of a cry due to pain. Mothers must learn to recognize the normal conversational cries of their children by close association from the time of birth.

Demand feeding has many advantages. It is obviously wrong to force a baby to take food into a stomach that is not demanding it, and, although many will do so, they are more predisposed to colic or spitting up than those who only accept a meal for which their stomach is ready.

Much crying in a frustrated baby is undoubtedly a greater evil than has been recognized in the past.* Violent crying deprives a child's brain of the full quota of oxygen that he would have in a restful state. Many babies cry very violently when they are annoyed by not having what their body obviously demands, and these fits of irritation can definitely do harm, not only to the child's personality, but also to his physical and mental development. The baby, and the baby only, feels when he is ready for nourishment, and a mother, feeding on demand, soon knows to within a few minutes the digestive cycle of her child.

BABY'S PERFECT FOOD

Mother's milk has certain qualities that cannot be exactly duplicated. It has been created specifically for the human baby's own digestive system. It develops within the child an immunity against certain diseases, infections, and tooth decay. In families that suffer from such allergic diseases as asthma, eczema or hives, infants who are entirely breastfed for the earlier months of their lives are less prone to develop these conditions.

Breastfeeding is easier for the mother, for the baby's milk is always fresh, clean, easily available, and at the correct temperature. It is also both economical and labor saving, for there is no need to waste time sterilizing bottles and preparing

* Margaret A. Ribble, *The Rights of Infants*, rev. ed. (New York: Columbia University Press, 1965).

food, or buying expensive prepackaged formula in bottles. It contains all the essential elements of food for the baby.

ROOMING-IN

The profound importance to the baby of the first forty-eight hours of its neonatal life does not receive the emphasis many of us wish it had. For my own part I extend that thought to the development of the mother in the first forty-eight hours of motherhood. A newborn baby should remain with the mother during this extremely important period, where she can constantly see him and attend to him if necessary, even from the first day.

Forty-five or fifty years ago nurseries for all newborn babies were hailed as one of the latest advances in maternity wards. Up until that time it was usual to have the babies in cots either attached to or standing beside the mother's bed. The change proved to be a most unfortunate divergence from what was then termed the "old-fashioned" principle of leaving the babies with their mothers. It arose because of the increased use of heavy anesthesia for the mother, who was then in no condition even to be aware of the presence of the child and might cause him harm before she awakened to consciousness. The babies also needed much more constant medical supervision because of their own sedated state and associated problems.

But in recent years several important factors have brought about a change, so that in many up-to-date hospitals rooming-in has been reestablished.* One of these factors is a recognition of the importance of the mother-child relationship and the emotional development of the baby during the first few days of

---

* *Standards for Obstetric-Gynecologic Hospital Services* (Chicago: The American College of Obstetricians and Gynecologists, 1969), pp. 14 f., 44 f.; *Standards and Recommendations for Hospital Care of Newborn Infants* (Evanston, Ill.: American Academy of Pediatrics, 1964), pp. 30–33, 77.

his life. A mother who has been alert and cooperative during the birth presents no danger to the newborn left under her watchful eye.

Unless stringent protective measures are constantly employed, devastating epidemic infections in hospital nurseries still threaten to occur, for these infections now resist the previously effective antibiotics. Infants kept with their own mothers escape the risk of infant-to-infant skin, intestinal, and respiratory infections.

The results of a long and intricate investigation of rooming-in by Harvey Carey of Auckland University have been published, along with a number of similar studies. He found that the mother was the safest person to handle the baby, his research demonstrating that the nursing staff could be a source of danger in spreading the lesions of the staphylococcus, even though uninfected themselves. Rooming-in means that as far as possible no one but the mother handles the baby. The additional great advantage is that the baby receives individual attention, is fed when necessary, and is made comfortable when required. Researches show that babies put on weight better under rooming-in and that the mother is more confident in handling her baby, even though she now leaves the hospital only a few days after the birth. And of course under these conditions breastfeeding also has a much better chance of being successful.

Editors' Addendum

INFANT CARE IN THE NURSERY*

1. For a nursing mother, the "normal" baby is to be given no supplements, either milk or water, unless requested by the attending physician and/or the mother of the baby. If during the night in the first twenty-four hours a nursing baby appears fussy and the mother is asleep, the mother is to be awakened to nurse her baby, unless the mother states or gives other instructions.
2. If the baby and mother are discharged home in the first twenty-four hours and the PKU test has not been performed, the mother must be given instructions to return to the laboratory the next day with the infant for this test.
3. Personnel wash their hands before and after handling each infant. Newborn infants are to be under unremitting observation for the presence of cyanosis, hemorrhage, jaundice, dyspnea, vomiting, dehydration and/or abnormal activity.
4. The first stool and urine is noted and recorded. An antiseptic is applied to the umbilical cord. Infant's temperature is measured on admission and every four hours until stabilized, and then once daily.
5. Each infant is weighed once daily.
6. On discharge, the nursery nurse discusses with the mother any questions or problems concerning the immediate home care of the baby and checks to be sure the mother has an appointment back to her attending physician for the follow-up care of the baby.
7. All placentas are to be tagged and saved for the first twenty-four hours. If at the end of this time there has been no request to send the placenta to the pathology laboratory, the placenta is disposed of in the usual manner.
8. The following list is to be considered a newborn critical list and requires pediatric consultation:
   a. Respirations above 60.

* See also Haire, Doris, *Implementing Family-Centered Maternity Care with a Central Nursery:* (CEA of New Jersey, 1968).

b. Persistent *cyanosis*.
c. Repeated vomiting first 48 hours.
d. Loss of more than 10 percent birthweight.
e. Absence of *meconium* in first bowel movement.
f. Abdominal distention.
g. Rectal temperature over 101° Fahrenheit.
h. Birthweight under four pounds eight ounces.
i. Viable infant with severe malformation.
j. Rh sensitization.
k. Jaundice in first twenty-four hours.

SUGGESTED ROOMING-IN PROCEDURES*

Keeping the newborn baby as close to the mother as long as possible on the first and second days of life is advantageous both to the mother and the baby, psychologically and physically. Nursing personnel should be trained to encourage and assist in accomplishing this type program, as efficiently as possible within the facilities available.

1. Immediately following birth and in the birth room, the baby is to be first placed in the warmer, which should be placed right next to the mother. As soon as the temperature has stabilized in the baby, the mother is encouraged to hold the baby and touch him, having previously cleansed her hands (as has the husband), and the new father is also encouraged to touch his baby or hold him.
2. If the mother desires to nurse on the birth table, this can be accomplished. Moving the hood of the warmer over the mother assures the warmth of the baby.
3. A scale should be in the birth room so the baby need not be taken to the nursery to be weighed, or his data recorded.
4. The baby in the warmer is to stay in the birth room as long as possible while the mother is being prepared to return to her ward bed.
5. The baby can then be taken to the nursery for any additional care, but as soon as it is convenient for the nursery staff, hope-

---

* See also *Standards and Recommendations for Hospital Care of Newborn Infants* (American Academy of Pediatrics, 1966), for both nursery procedures and guidance in rooming-in in American hospitals.

fully within the first hour, the baby will be returned to the mother and to the bassinette at her bedside. Many times the baby bypasses the nursery, going with his mother directly from the birth room to her postpartum room.

6. When there are no other patients in the room, it seems advisable for the baby to stay with the mother as much as possible and as long as she requests his presence.

7. When the baby is in the room with the mother, the only visitors permitted will be the husband, who must be properly gowned, capped and masked. The infant's mother and father are the only two people in the world with whom he is bacteriologically compatible.

8. If other visitors are to visit the postpartum patient who has a rooming-in baby, the baby must be returned to the nursery while the visitors are present.

9. It is an important part of the staff's responsibility to take time whenever possible to help educate the new mother with as much information as possible for newborn baby care at home.

11

The New Mother

After the natural birth of a child a healthy woman need not remain in bed for more than two or three days. No mother should become bedridden after childbirth. Unless there is any definite contraindication, which the medical attendant will judge, she can be out of bed for short periods of time on the day her baby is born. On the second day she can be up a little more. Any feeling of tiredness is the signal that she has been up long enough, and she should rest as soon as she feels the need. The upright position and the exercises she does after the baby is born have many advantages.

The immediate adoption of good posture is important. So many women walk about after labor as if they had been seriously ill for a month; we see them in maternity hospitals after an uncomplicated birth stooping, hanging onto someone's arm, and staggering rather than walking. This postnatal assumption of illness is, in most cases, a psychological demand for activity, and an entirely uncalled-for condition in a healthy woman who has been properly cared for. She should be a happy, upright, easy-moving person glowing with the bloom of health, and with the expression of happiness on her face that is the prerogative of young mothers.

A certain amount of sensible discretion must be used when the mother arrives home with her new baby, and her husband or other helpers should take over her regular household chores for a week or ten days so she can devote her full attention to her baby without becoming weary or discouraged. At the end of six weeks she should revisit her physician.

AFTERPAINS

Women who have had more than one baby may have painful contractions of the uterus for the first day or two after the baby is born. Sometimes these are very slight, occurring especially when the baby is put to the breast. This is due to the reflex stimulation of the uterus from the breast, which makes it contract tightly during nursing, and assists in the rapid restoration of the uterus to its nonpregnant state.

Relaxation does not always relieve the pain, for it may spring from a different cause than in labor. If these contractions are severe enough to hurt, it probably means that there is a small blood clot or piece of membrane that has not yet come away from the uterine cavity. Many women resign themselves to these afterpains, which is wrong. If this discomfort arises they should say so immediately, for there is no reason why they should not be relieved of it very quickly. A mild pain reliever such as one quarter grain of codeine followed by two tablets of aspirin four hours later usually works like a charm, and the discomfort probably will not recur.

LOCHIA

For two weeks or even longer after labor, a discharge persists from the genital canal. This discharge, or *lochia,* is largely composed of the debris of the uterine and vaginal walls as they cast off those membranes and tissues which were of service during pregnancy and birth. It consists largely of thin blood with a few small clots and, in three or four days, turns a brownish color. Apart from frequent cleansing and the wearing of sanitary napkins, this should occasion no more inconvenience than rather prolonged menstruation.

CARE OF THE NIPPLES

The nipples must be kept soft and elastic. They should be cleansed with warm water only, for even soap has a drying effect. The application of chemicals with the intention of making them hard and strong does more harm than good and predisposes to cracking and sore places. The nipples should be made to stand out so that nursing is easy for the baby; this can be done by proper care during the last weeks of pregnancy, as described earlier (page 150).* Sore nipples should be exposed to the air for fifteen minutes after nursing. A cream such as Nivea is soothing.

If milk has to be expressed from the breast after nursing has been established, the expelling movement is the same as that used in preparation of the nipple. The left hand used for the right breast and the right hand for the left breast, the base of the brown area should be pressed gently between the thumb and forefinger. The breasts should be relieved in this way of a little milk whenever they become uncomfortably full and it is not time to nurse the baby, to prevent painful engorgement. Gradually the amount of milk produced will adjust to the amount the baby requires.

BREASTFEEDING

Every mother should feed her baby at the breast. The advantages to the baby are often mentioned, but it is equally important to the mother's health and emotional well-being. It consolidates the mother-child relationship from the earliest hours of birth. The breastfeeding mother is conscious of a

---

* A variety of breast shields are available that are helpful in overcoming such problems as inverted nipples, weak suckling as in a premature infant, or sore nipples. These problems should be under the physician's care and advice.

satisfying sense of achievement when her baby is at the breast. The close contact and physical stimulus of the baby's suckling bring nearer to her mind the reality of motherhood, its joys, and its responsibilities. We must not overlook the importance of the daydreams of a nursing mother. Not infrequently a new outlook upon life is developed that brings a serenity of mind, enhancing for all time the patience and self-control so necessary in the upbringing and training of children.

Nursing the child not only assists the uterus and birth canal in returning to their normal shape and size, but it also releases into the mother's bloodstream chemicals that have a tranquilizing effect upon her, once breastfeeding is well established. Before that time, consciously relaxing will help the breast "let down" the milk. The problem in breastfeeding is not the supply, but the "giving" of the milk. A tense mother inhibits the "let-down" reflex of her milk, so that both she and the baby become frustrated. When she has learned to relax well enough to allow the milk to flow as the baby nurses, the stimulation to her system will result in still further calmness and pleasure.

A mother breastfeeding her baby must be in a comfortable position so that she can relax well, and avoid any strain on her back and shoulder muscles. Many women sit hunched up with their heads dropping forward to watch the baby anxiously, only to find that in a short time their backs are aching from the neck to the waist. It is best to sit in a high-backed chair with a pillow across the knees and the baby lying on the pillow, its head level with the nipples. The mother puts one arm around the child and lets its head rest on her forearm. With the other hand she gently depresses the breast from under the baby's nose to give him a free airway.

If she prefers to lie in bed, the baby can lie beside her. This is not only comfortable but enables the baby to take the nipple into his mouth without dragging on the breast.

It should be remembered that if an infant is fed from below, with the nipple pulled downward into his mouth, after three or four months the shape of the breast may be irreparably damaged. Thus, if a mother wants to keep her attractive physical shape, the correct position for nursing is important.

Let me offer this solace to the woman who would, but cannot, feed her baby at the breast. She will find this disappointment can lead to a deep and cherished bond that turns the water of weaning into the wine of spiritual communion. A gypsy mother, whose breasts had been incurably mutilated by the flames of an exploding stove, was feeding her fifth baby from a bottle. She had breastfed the four beautiful children who ran to greet me. They were clean, friendly, and lovable in their picturesque, highly colored clothes and gilded earrings. I sat in the spotless caravan and told her how grieved I was to have to suppress her milk flow. "Don't worry, doctor," she told me. "It's all the same if you put your heart into the bottle."

If a mother must bottle-feed her baby, let her give him the milk herself, with warmth, love, and security, snuggled to her heart in the silent serenity of mutual satisfaction. It is well to let the baby snuggle "skin-to-skin" against her breast as he nurses from the bottle. Then little will be lost and much will be recovered.

ROOMING-IN

Many mothers suffer silent acute anxiety for the welfare of their babies during the first three or four days of life if the baby is in some place apart. But if it remains in the room with her, she will see the nurse change the baby's diapers and oil its skin, for newborn babies are not bathed with water and soap for the first few days. She will learn what his different cries mean and will gain confidence in her ability to care for her child, under the supervision of the nursing staff. This closeness to the infant, so that he can be fed on demand any time of the day or night, stimulates early and efficient breastfeeding, often before the mother leaves the hospital.

It is not correct to say that the presence of a baby is disturbing to a mother and does not enable her to have sufficient rest. The baby that is "roomed-in" with his mother is very rarely restless, and the mother who wishes to have her baby with her is almost invariably at peace with herself and the world.

DIET

The same principles of good diet apply during breast-feeding as during pregnancy. The nursing mother should continue to take two pints of milk a day, and drink more water than before the baby was born. Apart from that, she should eat sensibly, simply, and discreetly, recognizing the essential constituents of food and including them in sufficient, but not excessive, amounts to maintain good health and provide for the development of the baby. She should look upon meals as important and pleasant pauses in the daily round, eat slowly, enjoying the natural flavors of food, for quality is of more pleasure than quantity, and should stop before feeling full. She should be restful and relaxed in comfort and conversation, stop before feeling full, and should spend fifteen minutes in quiet reading or rest before returning to the duties of the day. This aids digestion and prevents the signs and symptoms of avoidable indigestion.

POSTNATAL EXERCISES

The objects of postnatal exercises are:

1. To promote efficient circulation of the blood.
2. To maintain the habit of full and controlled breathing learned during the prenatal training.
3. To regain good posture and carriage.
4. To aid the absorption and natural distribution of fat stored in and on the body during pregnancy.
5. To restore the firmness and muscle tone of the abdominal and pelvic muscles.

The average mother does not have much time for exercises

and relaxation, especially if she has one or two other children to care for. She will be less tired, however, and more efficient if she organizes her daily routine so that a quarter of an hour is spent on these few exercises, followed by fifteen to thirty minutes of deep relaxation.

Breathing

Deep, full breathing should be begun on the second day. It is enough to take *six full, controlled breaths three times during the day*.

Firming the Pelvic Floor

It is extremely important that the muscles and tissues of the pelvis, which have been stretched and considerably loosened during childbirth, should be restored to their normal tone and strength. Many of the discomforts that follow childbirth are due to the absence of this care. This exercise should be done on the second day after the arrival of the baby, and continued for the rest of the mother's life. It is the same exercise as exercise 5 in the prenatal instructions.

Tightly squeeze together the muscles of the vulva and vagina, much more firmly than the effort required when there is a desire to urinate at an inconvenient moment. This "squeezing up" need not be associated in any way with movements of the thighs or buttocks. After tightening these muscles, hold them tight for a moment when the tension is greatest, and then relax them slowly. This has the effect of drawing up the pelvic floor, tightening the ring around and within the vaginal orifice, and closing firmly the small tube through which urine is passed. This should be done *twelve times, two or three times a day*.

Firming the Abdominal Muscles

On the third day after the arrival of the baby, after taking a few full, deep breaths, lying on the back, raise the left knee up to the chest, with the knee bent. Straighten the leg and lower it slowly onto the bed. Repeat with the right leg. Do this with each leg once or twice the first day, gradually increasing to *five or six times once a day*.

Firming the Breasts

This is the same as prenatal exercise 4. Grip each arm firmly behind the wrist and raise the arms to the level of the shoulders. Push the skin of the forearm up while tightening the arm muscles and the muscles of the chest, lifting the breasts. Release the tension slowly, so the breasts do not drop suddenly. Repeat *ten times, once a day*. It is especially important to continue this exercise during weaning, to keep the muscle support of the breasts in good tone.

Pelvic Rock*

This is the same as prenatal exercise 1. On hands and knees, let the back sag. Slowly raise the back, at the same time squeezing together the muscles of the buttocks, pelvic area, and upper legs.

Conclusion

After completing the exercises, a period of relaxation should follow, lying on the abdomen with the legs extended, or in the lateral side position as in pregnancy and labor. These positions take the weight of the still bulky uterus off the pelvic floor and help to prevent it from falling backward and down toward the pelvis as it returns to normal size.

I advise women to exaggerate their posture for the first few days, pulling the abdomen well in and the hips under, and

---

* The arms must be kept extended during this exercise, with the elbows straight, so that the chest is not lower than the hips. The "knee-chest" position sometimes prescribed for postpartum patients is to be avoided, as it causes air to be sucked into the vagina, and may create an air embolism in the bloodstream.

"standing tall," with shoulders back and head and chin up. Breathe in such a manner that the chest expands and fills the hollows below the collarbones. This slight exaggeration of posture enables rapid reabsorption to take place in the softened connective tissue around the pelvic joints and lower spine, with the minimum risk of discomfort from backache.

Relaxation must be persisted in, for it is of great advantage in successful breastfeeding. If the mother has opportunity for relaxation as she nurses her baby, does her breathing and other exercises, and persists throughout her life in the habitual performance of the pelvic tensing and relaxing, she will be laying the foundation of good health and happiness for herself, as well as efficient breastfeeding of her newborn infant.